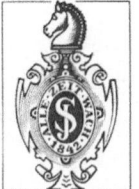

A. Huber A.H.C.v. Hochstetter M. Allgöwer

Transsphincteric Surgery of the Rectum

Topographical Anatomy and Operation Technique

With 31 Figures, Most in Color, in 58 Separate Illustrations

Springer-Verlag
Berlin Heidelberg NewYork Tokyo 1984

PD Dr. med. Andreas Huber
Chirurgische Klinik, Kantonsspital, CH-6004 Luzern

Prof. Dr. Arthur H.C. von Hochstetter
Leiter der Abteilung für topographische und klinische Anatomie,
Departement für Chirurgie, Kantonsspital, CH-4031 Basel
formerly: Professor of Anatomy at the University of Western
Ontario, London, Ontario, Canada

Prof. Dr. Martin Allgöwer
Departement für Chirurgie, Kantonsspital, CH-4031 Basel

Translator: Terry C. Telger, 3054 Vaughan Avenue, Marina,
CA 93933/USA

Title of the original German edition: *Transsphinktere Rektumchirurgie*
© Springer-Verlag Berlin Heidelberg New York Tokyo 1983
ISBN 3-540-12583-3 / 0-387-12583-3

ISBN-13: 978-3-642-69472-1   e-ISBN-13: 978-3-642-69470-7
DOI: 10.1007/978-3-642-69470-7

Library of Congress Cataloging in Publication Data. Huber, Andreas. Trans-
sphincteric surgery of the rectum. Translation of: Transsphinktere Rektumchirurgie.
Bibliography: p. Includes index. 1. Rectum-Surgery. 2. Anus-Surgery. I. Hochstetter,
A.H.C.v. (Arthur H.C.), 1918 –. II. Allgöwer, M. (Martin), 1917 –. III. Title.
(DNLM: 1. Rectum-Surgery. WI 650 H877t) RD544.H813 1984 617'.555 83-20268

2124/3140-543210

Foreword

More than a century ago, Cripps successfully employed the direct and complete division of the anal sphincters as a means of approaching the lower rectum and anal canal, and reported on a series of 36 patients who had been treated in that fashion. Cripps was pleasantly surprised to find good fecal continence in over two-thirds of the patients during later follow-ups, despite the fact that the divided sphincters had not been repaired. The transsphincteric procedure was largely forgotten in subsequent years, however, and only the parasacral proctotomy of Kraske, which spared the anal sphincters, can be said to have gained an established place in the "surgical armamentarium."

It remained for York Mason to redirect the attention of the surgical community to the great potential of the transsphincteric approach and the excellent continence that can be achieved through adequate repair of the divided sphincters. Having recognized the outstanding practical value of this procedure, we felt it necessary to define more precisely the anatomical prerequisites that would ensure minimum operative bleeding, and to bring the procedure more in line with current knowledge of normal continence and defecation.

Dr. A. Huber, in consultation with the director of the Institute for Clinical Anatomy of our surgical department, Prof. A. von Hochstetter, did many months of dissection work on fresh anatomic preparations in an effort to explore and refine the various aspects of the transsphincteric approach. During this time his discoveries were repeatedly tested for clinical relevance in patients suffering from rectal disease. The present, short monograph details the experience and insights that have been gained from this process.

The major indications for the transsphincteric, "open-book" procedure are benign but refractory rectal diseases such as rectovaginal fistulae, benign ulcers, villous adenomas, marked rectal prolapses, and selected cases of marked rectocele. In the latter condition in particular, it is advantageous to combine an extensive sleeve resection of the rectum with reefing of the puborectalis sling to modify the anorectal angle. If adequate ventilation is maintained in the prone patient, the 2- to 3-hour operation is remarkably well tolerated even by aged individuals.

In the case of rectal malignancies, the procedure should be limited to growths which have not spread beyond the rectal wall (UICC $T_1N_2N_0$ or Dukes Type A). But the "sacred cow" of a 5-cm distal wall clearance may at last be dispensed with. The fate of a rectal carcinoma hinges on its pararectal spread, and a safety margin of 2 cm is generally sufficient for wall resections. Thus, *small* growths less than 3 cm in diameter that are confined to the bowel wall may be removed by a sphincter-conserving resection up to 5 cm from the anocutaneous junction, relying upon frozen tissue sections to monitor the adequacy of the resection.

We personally are very pleased with this addition to our surgical arsenal and hope that it will be equally useful and successful in other hands.

Basel, September 1983   Martin Allgöwer

Table of Contents

Part I
Transsphincteric Surgery
of the Rectum

1. Significance

Surgical removal of diseased tissue from the lower rectum, or the resection of this bowel segment, calls for a highly refined operating technique. This is due mainly to the close proximity and attachments that the lower rectum has with the pelvic floor muscles and the anal sphincters. Together, the rectum, pelvic floor and sphincters comprise an organ system whose function is to ensure normal defecation and anal continence. The challenge to the surgeon is to cure disease in this hard-to-reach area without destroying fecal continence. Transsphincteric exposure of the rectum is a technique which is compatible with this goal. Applied selectively, this procedure offers an excellent chance of a cure without forcing the patient to accept a "preternatural anus."

The idea of a transsphincteric approach to the rectum is not new. Various authors had already outlined its basic features by the latter part of the 19th Century. In 1875 Verneuil and Kocher described a posterior exposure of the rectum which required a coccygectomy, and in 1885 Kraske recommended that partial resection of the left ala of the sacrum be added to this procedure. In 1876 Cripps published an essay on the transsphincteric approach to the rectum and reported on 36 patients whose rectal tumors had been removed by that technique. It is interesting to note that, although Cripps made no attempt to suture the divided sphincters, 23 of the 36 patients regained full fecal continence following surgery. Although numerous references were made to this procedure in subsequent years (Bevan 1917; David 1943; Larkin 1959; Oh and Kark 1972), a great many surgeons were reluctant to adopt it, apparently in the belief that division of the levator ani and sphincters would result in permanent anal incontinence. More recently, Mason (1974) published an account of his left parasacral transsphincteric exposure and the excellent results he achieved with it. Since that report, we have been practicing the Mason technique of transsphincteric rectal surgery at the Kantonsspital Basel, Switzerland, and have obtained equally good results.

We feel that the transsphincteric approach will assume an increasingly important place in the anorectal surgery of the future. Given the strict criteria for patient selection, however, it is unlikely that this operation will become routine, at least in the general surgical hospital. Moreover, the pelvis and pelvic floor possess a highly complex and variable anatomy. For example, we have observed large individual differences in the mass and arrangement of the levator ani muscle, as well as in the "perirectal space," which frequently contains a large amount of fat permeated with delicate blood vessels that are highly prone to injury. In the literature on transsphincteric rectal surgery, anatomical aspects usually are discussed only in highly simplified terms, and questions relating to anatomical details such as the innervation of the pelvic floor frequently go unanswered. In an effort to fill this gap, we have created a combined surgical and anatomical atlas in which a special section has been devoted to the topographic anatomy of the anorectal region.

2. Definition

Transsphincteric surgery of the rectum refers to procedures in which exposure of the terminal bowel segment is gained through a posterior division of the pelvic floor, possibly combined with an anal sphincterotomy. During the operation the patient is prone with the legs slightly abducted and the hip and knee joints flexed 90° (the Heidelberg position). Through a left parasacral incision, the pelvic floor is opened, and, if necessary, the sphincters are divided so that the distal portion of the rectum and anal canal can be visualized. At the conclusion of the procedure the pelvic floor and sphincters are anatomically repaired so that normal defecation and continence are preserved.

3. Indications

Disease

The following diseases of the rectum and anal canal are considered to be indications for transsphincteric surgery:

- Early, low-sited rectal malignancies which are not amenable to a low anterior resection.
- Benign and premalignant tumors which cannot be radically removed by the transanal route.
- Rectal prolapse with incontinence.
- Rectal fistulae and strictures which cannot be managed by any other method.
- Lesions of the pelvic floor and sphincters.
- Malformations.

Indications are discussed in greater detail in Part IV.

Localization

The site of the lesion is another important criterion for patient selection. The transsphincteric approach is best suited for lesions located between 4 and 12 cm from the anal verge. Complete division of the sphincters extends the operative field caudally to the pectinate line. Under favorable circumstances, cranial portions of the rectosigmoid located up to 30 cm from the anal verge can be reached by the transsphincteric route. If this approach does not allow adequate cranial mobilization (which is unlikely with careful preoperative planning), then a laparotomy will also be required. Turning the patient to the supine position and back to the Heidelberg position is somewhat cumbersome but should not cause serious difficulties if proper precautions are taken.

Patients

The Heidelberg position is surprisingly well tolerated even by aged and debilitated patients. Assuming that anesthesia is correctly administered, there need be no hesitation in selecting these patients for transsphincteric surgery. The operation lasts about $2^1/_2$ hours on the average and apparently is less stressful than a laparotomy, for example.

4. Preoperative Preparation

As in any surgical procedure, patient selection, preoperative preparation and post-operative care have a critical bearing on the success of the operation.

Preoperative preparations include the thorough cleansing of the colorectum, preferably by an intestinal lavage of the type generally recommended for colonic surgery. If the passage of fecal matter is significantly impaired by rectal disease, then a three-stage procedure employing a temporary colostomy is advised. We administer prophylactic antibiotics shortly before and during the operation. This is an effective means of preventing infection, provided sufficiently high serum levels are present at the time of operation.

An operating table must be made available which allows the patient to be placed in the Heidelberg position. The table setup, the Heidelberg position, and preparation of the operative field are described in Part III.

5. Postoperative Care

The transsphincteric operation is excellently tolerated, and early ambulation is encouraged. Oral nutrition may be started as soon as bowel motility has resumed – usually on about the second postoperative day. Enemas are to be avoided, but mineral oil preparations may be given orally to aid bowel movements.

6. Follow-up Examinations

Regular follow-up examinations should be scheduled for the purpose of monitoring surgical wound healing and testing for continence. Examinations for healing are especially important following the removal of malignant growths and may be conducted as a part of general oncologic aftercare. While the bowel lumen is accessible to inspection through a proctoscope, computerized tomography is the best technique for evaluating the pararectal space, allowing the very early detection of recurrent growths and local metastases.

Postoperative continence is assessed on the basis of subjective reports and objective findings (manometry). It may require weeks or even months to develop, especially following the transsphincteric resection of a rectal prolapse with reefing of the puborectalis sling and a "posterior release" (Fig. 1, pp. 8/9). Particular attention should be given to subjective reports on continence for flatus and for liquid and formed stool at rest as well as during coughing, sneezing, and other acts which raise the intra-abdominal pressure. The tone and voluntary function of the external sphincter and levator ani can be assessed by rectal palpation.

7. Complications

Complications are rare. Patients who were continent preoperatively will regain continence within a few weeks after surgery. If incontinence is present preoperatively, it often is markedly improved by reefing and posterior release of the levator slings and, with rectal prolapse, by resection of the prolapsed bowel. If there is already severe preexisting damage to the pelvic floor, there is no guarantee that surgery will be of value in improving continence. The attempt should nevertheless be made, however, because surgery can only help the situation and cannot harm it.

Postoperative wound infection is rare if the bowel has been thoroughly cleansed prior to surgery, a suitable operating technique was employed, and prophylactic antibiotics have been administered. Infection can cause dehiscence of the sutures in the pelvic floor muscles and sphincters, leading to incontinence. Treatment for an extensive wound infection includes broad exposure and drainage of the wound, and the establishment of a temporary colostomy. After the infection has resolved, it should be possible to repair the pelvic floor secondarily and restore anal continence.

If infection arises from a gap in the suture line used for a rectal anastomosis and remains confined to a fistulous tract, there is little risk that continence will be damaged. The drained infection will heal if the rectum is kept empty for a time, either by making a temporary colostomy or by feeding an "astronaut" diet.

8. Remarks on Continence

Continence refers to the voluntary and involuntary control of defecation. A distinction may be made between gross and fine continence, where gross continence is the ability to control the voiding of large, solid feces, and fine continence is the control of small fecal masses, liquid feces and flatus. Thus, varying degrees of fecal incontinence may be present. Incontinence is said to be complete when the patient has no control whatsoever over the expulsion of feces or flatus.

Continence is maintained by a complex organ system comprised of the following elements:

- The rectum, the pelvic floor muscles (most notably the puborectalis sling), and the internal and external sphincters.
- The sensory and motor functions of these organs.
- Reflexes and central nervous mechanisms.

The following factors in this system contribute to continence:

The curvatures of the rectum in the frontal and sagittal planes and its transverse folds (Houston, Kohlrausch) retard progression of the fecal mass. Of particular importance is the anorectal angulation, whose function can be likened to that of a flutter valve or the phenomenon of a kinked garden hose. The anorectal angle is maintained by the pull of the puborectalis sling and by the anococcygeal ligament.

The stellate cross-section of the anal canal mucosa and its corpus cavernosum-like elements (hemorrhoidal plexus) are believed to exercise a sealing function.

The pressure that can be measured within the anal canal at rest results from the resting tone of the internal and external sphincters and the puborectalis muscle. It normally ranges between 30 cm H_2O (2.94 kPa) and 50 cm H_2O (4.9 kPa). With this pressure, the anal canal creates an effective barrier against the pressure of 10–30 cm H_2O (0.98–2.94 kPa) that resides within the rectum. Distension of the rectum reflexly triggers a transitory relaxation of the internal sphincter, accompanied by a measurable pressure fall within the anal canal. This makes possible the "sampling response" which enables rectal contents to be discriminated and their elimination controlled.

Voluntary contraction of the external sphincters can strengthen the barrier effect by increasing the pressure in the anal canal. This voluntary "squeeze pressure" can be sustained for only about a minute, however.

A rise of intra-abdominal pressure stimulates an increase in the tone of the external sphincters and puborectalis. This mechanism helps to maintain continence during coughing, sneezing and laughing.

A gradual increase in rectal distension produces a corresponding rise of pressure within the anal canal up to a level of 80–130 cm H_2O (7.84–12.74 kPa) (the "resting yield pressure"). Further distension of the rectum stimulates a voluntary contraction of the sphincters, raising the pressure as high as 400 cm H_2O (39.2 kPa) (the "augmented yield pressure"). One function of this reflex increase in voluntary sphincter contraction may be to preserve continence during sleep. At the same time, the compliant walls of the rectum expand in response to the elevated pressure or increasing mass, thus performing a reservoir function which also contributes to continence. This adaptive response is abolished by low rectal resections, but apparently it can be acquired to some degree by the bowel segment above the anastomosis. It is dependent, moreover, on a functionally-sound sphincter apparatus. Stretching of the external sphincters and the puborectalis sling excites the urge to defecate and triggers a voluntary contraction of these muscles. Two empirical facts are of great interest in this regard:

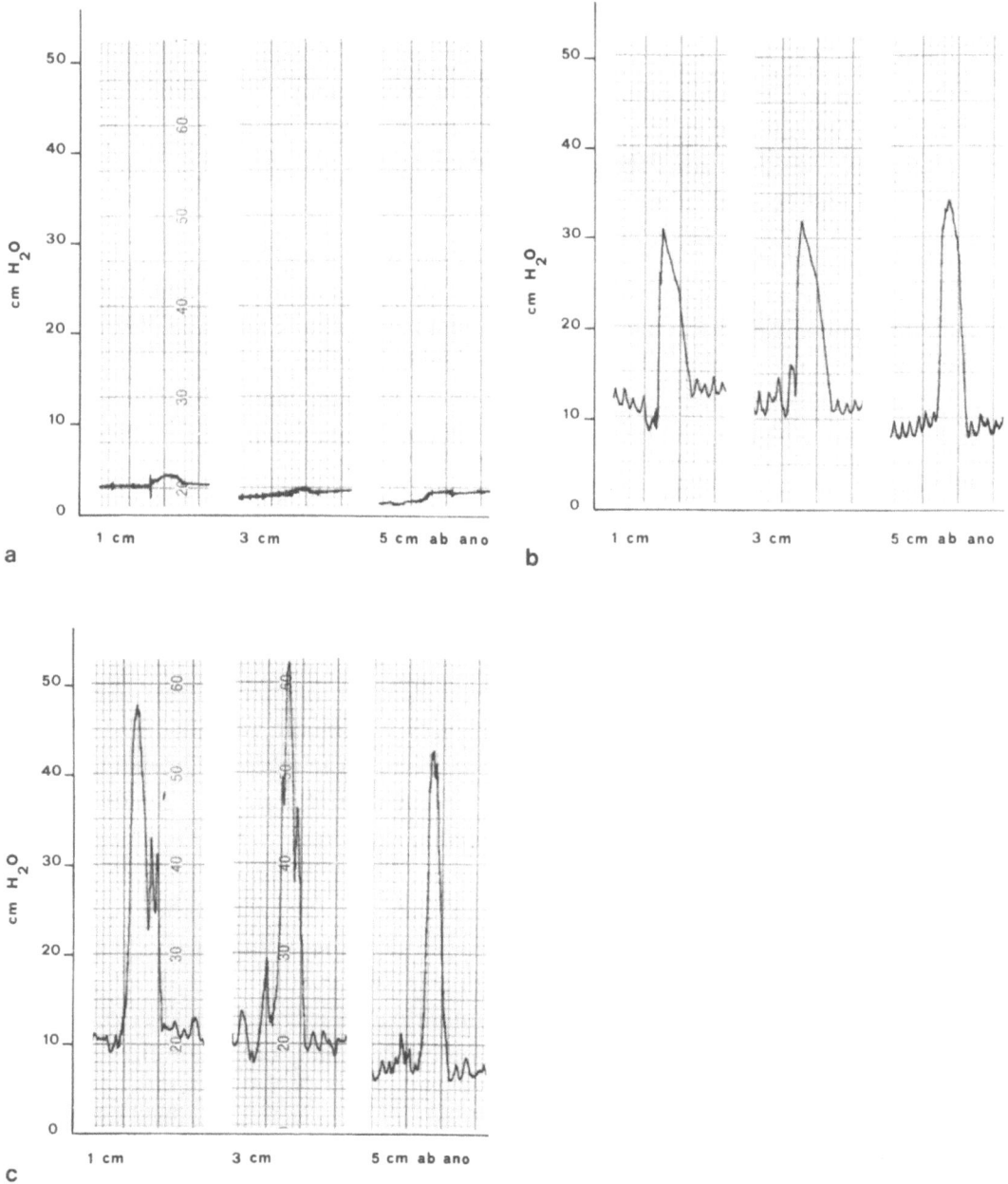

Fig. 1a–d. Manometric curves* of an 82-year-old woman who underwent transsphincteric surgery for rectal prolapse with incontinence. The pressures were measured with open-tipped perfusion-pressure catheters, and closed rectal balloons were used to induce distension. The curves were traced from right to left at a rate of 5 cm/min. The zero baseline and pressure values correspond to the numbers on the ordinate, not those on the record paper.

* M. Durig, M.D., Department of Surgery, Kantonsspital Basel, Switzerland: Personal communication

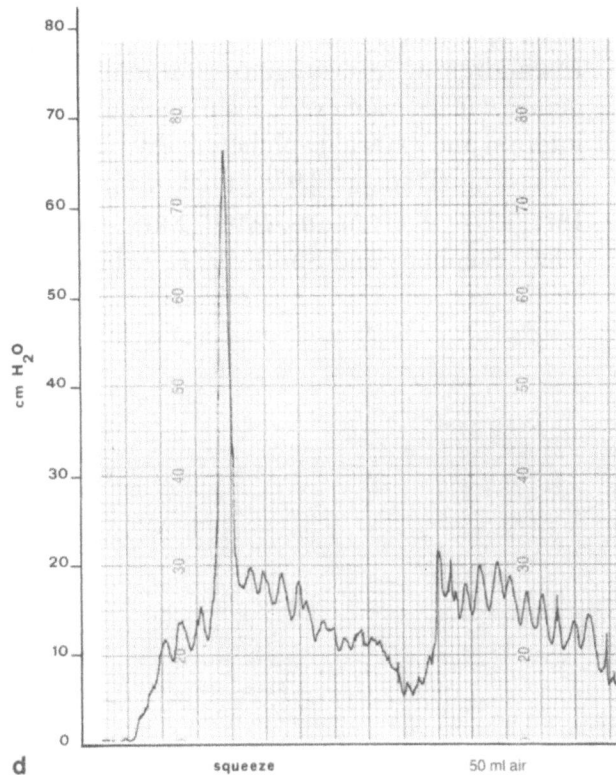

d   squeeze   50 ml air

a Preoperatively the resting pressure in the anal canal was about 3 cm H_2O (0.29 kPa) and showed little increase on voluntary squeezing of the sphincters.

b The rectal prolapse was resected through the transsphincteric approach, the puborectalis sling was reefed, and a posterior release was performed. A 30-cm segment of rectum was resected. Thus, the entire pars pelvina of the rectum was removed, and the "neorectum" consisted of sigmoid colon. One week postoperatively the resting pressure in the anal canal was 12 cm H_2O. Voluntary squeezing of the sphincters produced pressures of around 30 cm H_2O (2.95 kPa).

c At six weeks postoperatively (cf. **d**) the pressure was approximately 10 cm H_2O at rest (0.98 kPa) and up to 65 cm H_2O (6.37 kPa) on voluntary sphincter contraction.

d Distension of the neorectum reflexly triggered a brief relaxation of the internal sphincter like that seen during physiologic distension of the rectum. Following the pressure fall, a very strong rise of pressure was recorded. This is the "squeeze pressure" produced by voluntary contraction of the sphincters, which halts the propulsive wave in the rectum and can maintain continence for a short time.

1. Loss of the voluntary sphincter muscles, especially the puborectalis, results in complete incontinence.
2. In children with severe anorectal malformations, an acceptable degree of continence can be achieved, even in the absence of the rectum, anal canal, and internal and external sphincters, by pulling bowel through a functional puborectalis sling (Deucher 1976; Dickinson 1978; Goligher 1980; Harris et al. 1966; Ihre 1974; Kerremans 1969; Lane and Parks 1977; Scharli 1981; Shepherd 1980; Stephens and Smith 1971; Telander et al., in press; Wilson 1977).

Part II
Topographical Anatomy

Foundamentals and Methods

All illustrations (Figs. 2–14) are based upon specimens prepared at the Institute of Topographic and Clinical Anatomy of the Department of Surgery of the University of Basel. Working with von Hochstetter, specimens were selected, prepared, and then utilized to work out the relevant details of transsphincteric surgery.

The vivid anatomy of these preparations helped to provide much new information on the transsphincteric approach to the rectum and has prompted corresponding refinements of operating technique. In the present atlas, the technique of the transsphincteric approach as developed in collaboration with M. Allgöwer is extensively illustrated and described. It has proved its value in practice at our hospital.

All illustrations and schematic diagrams were prepared by A. Huber. The figures relating to topographic anatomy and operative technique were drawn with charcoal, and the schematic diagrams with ink. With one exception, coloring was done on photographic reproductions of the original drawings.

Work on the anatomic specimens is documented with photographs prepared at our center.

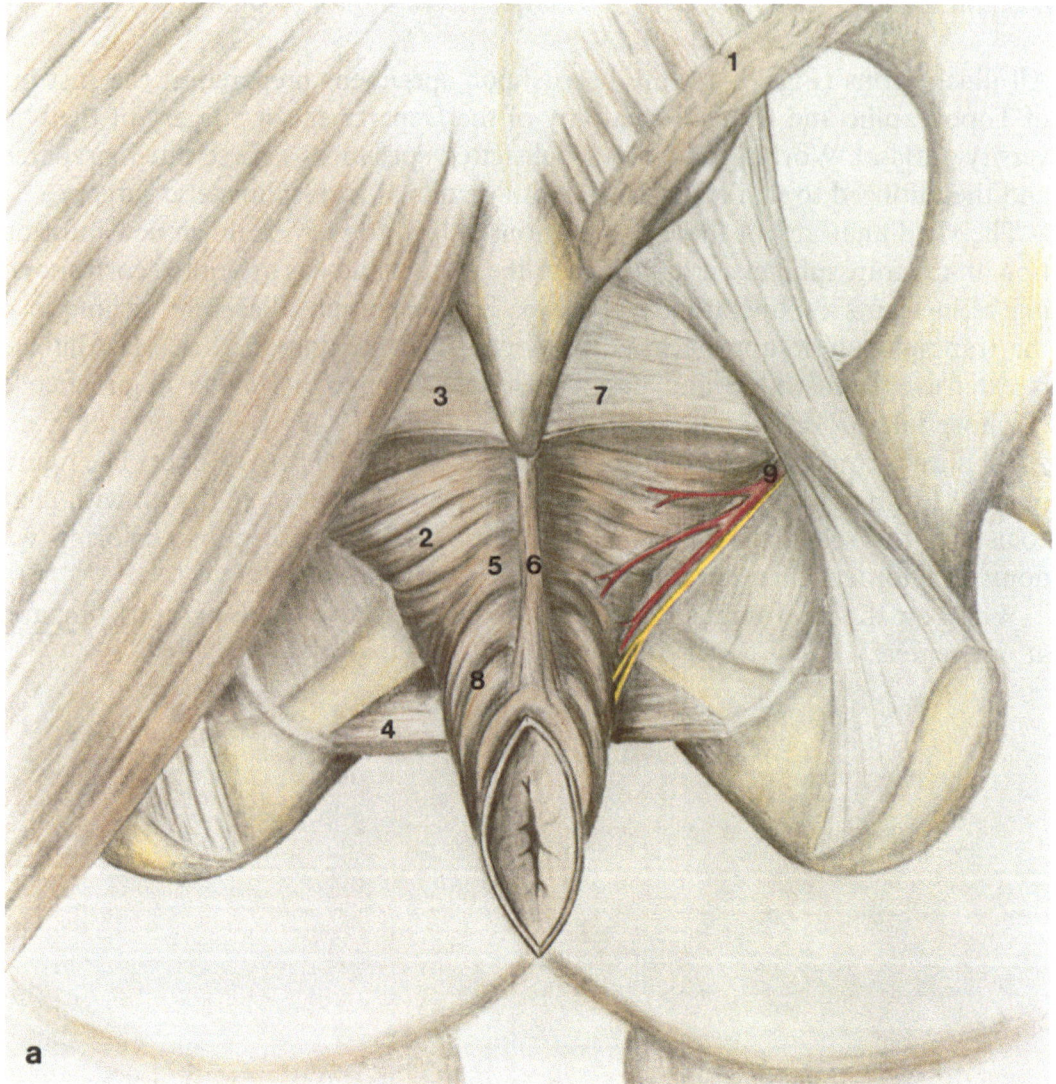

Fig. 2a, b. Preparation of a female pelvis. The posterior and slightly cranial view corresponds approximately to the viewpoint of a surgeon doing transsphincteric surgery on a patient in the Heidelberg position. The right gluteus maximus (*1*) is removed to better demonstrate the pelvic floor anatomy. We subdivide the pelvic floor, or pelvic diaphragm, into a rectal part and a urogenital part. The rectal diaphragm is formed by the two levator ani muscles (*2*) and the cocygeus muscles (*3*), and the urogenital diaphragm (*4*) by the deep and superficial perineus muscles.

The two levator muscles form a funnel whose outlet begins at the level of the puborectalis sling (*5*) and there angles sharply backward. The levator ani may be divided into three parts according to the origin of the fibers: a pubic part, a tendinous part, and an ischial part. The muscle arises anteriorly from the inner surface of the pubic bone (pubic part), more posteriorly from the inner

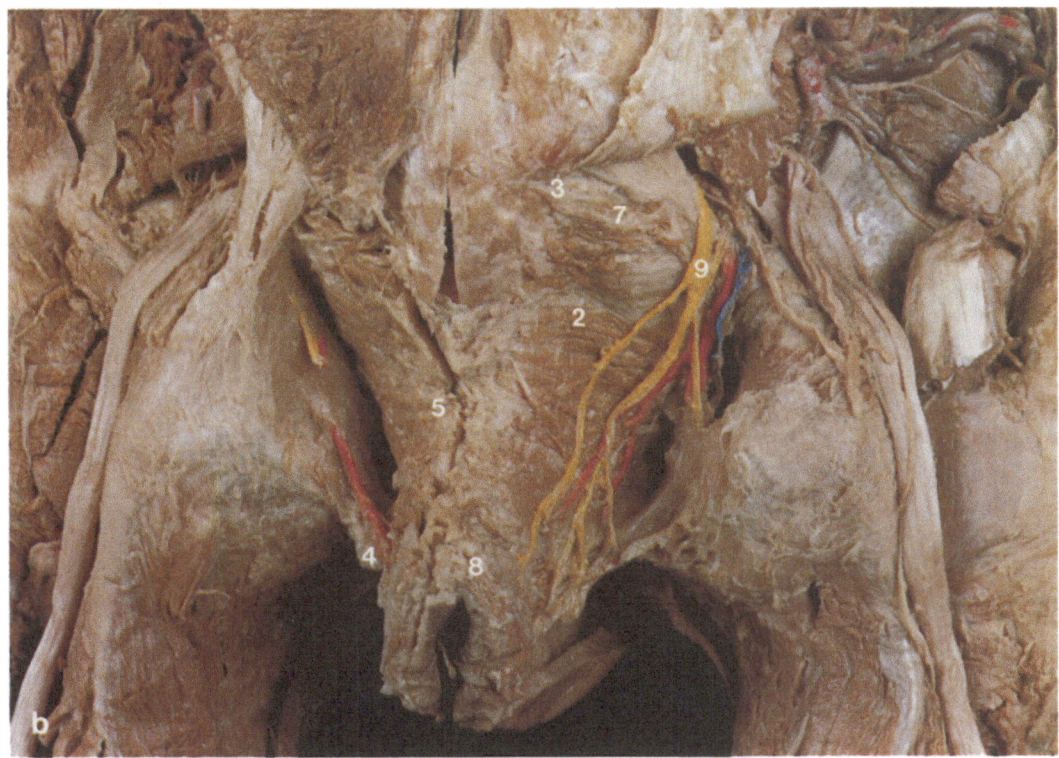

pelvic wall along the tendinous arch of the internal obturator fascia (tendinous part), and posteriorly from the ischial spine (ischial part). The medial fibers of the levator ani form a muscular sling which arises from the pubic bone and encircles the anorectal flexure. This structure, called the puborectalis sling (5), plays a crucial role in maintaining fecal continence. Posteriorly the two limbs of levator ani join at the anococcygeal raphe, which attaches to the tip of the coccyx. Muscle fibers which arise from the tip of the coccyx and blend with fibers of the external sphincter form the anococcygeal ligament (6). A free passage exists between this ligament and the anococcygeal raphe. Anteriorly, the two limbs of the levator form the borders of the levator portal, which is divided by muscle fibers converging at the centrum tendineum into the rectal hiatus, through which the rectum passes, and the urogenital hiatus, which is perforated by the urogenital organs. The latter hiatus is covered externally by the urogenital diaphragm.

The coccygeus muscles pass from the coccyx to the ischiadic spine and form the posterior portion of the pelvic floor. The fibers of the coccygeus (3) blend intimately with the sacrospinous ligament (7), and both are regarded as a structural unit. The size, arrangement and course of the levator ani and coccygeus muscles show a high degree of variability. The sphincter ani externus muscle (8) forms the lower part of the funnel of the pelvic floor (i.e., its outlet). It consists of three parts: subcutaneous, superficial, and deep.

The levator ani and sphincter ani externus are supplied with blood by branches (9) of the pudendal artery.

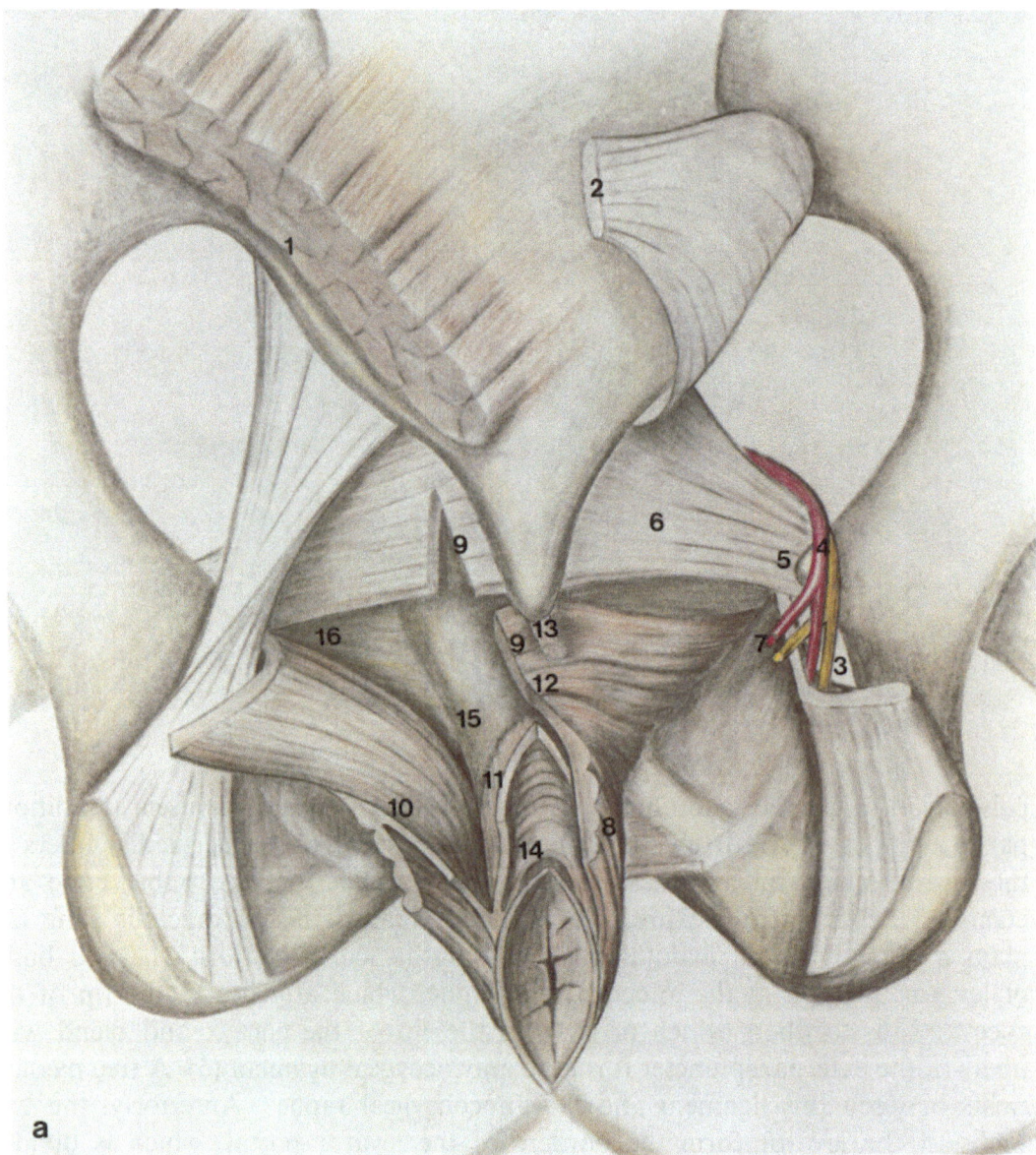

a

Fig. 3a, b. Additional dissection was done on the specimen in Fig. 1 to provide the model for this drawing. The left gluteus maximus (*1*) is removed, the right is not shown. The right sacrotuberous ligament (*2*) is divided and reflected upward

---

Fig. 2a, b *(continued)*

The nerve branch which arises from the pudendal nerve (*9*) supplies only the sphincter ani externus and the caudal part of the puborectalis. The levator ani and cranial part of the puborectalis are supplied by nerves from the sacral plexus which course on the inner surface of the pelvic floor. The rectal diaphragm is covered both internally and externally by fasciae which blend together at the levator portal. On the inner surface, the fascia is continuous with the internal parietal pelvic fascia.

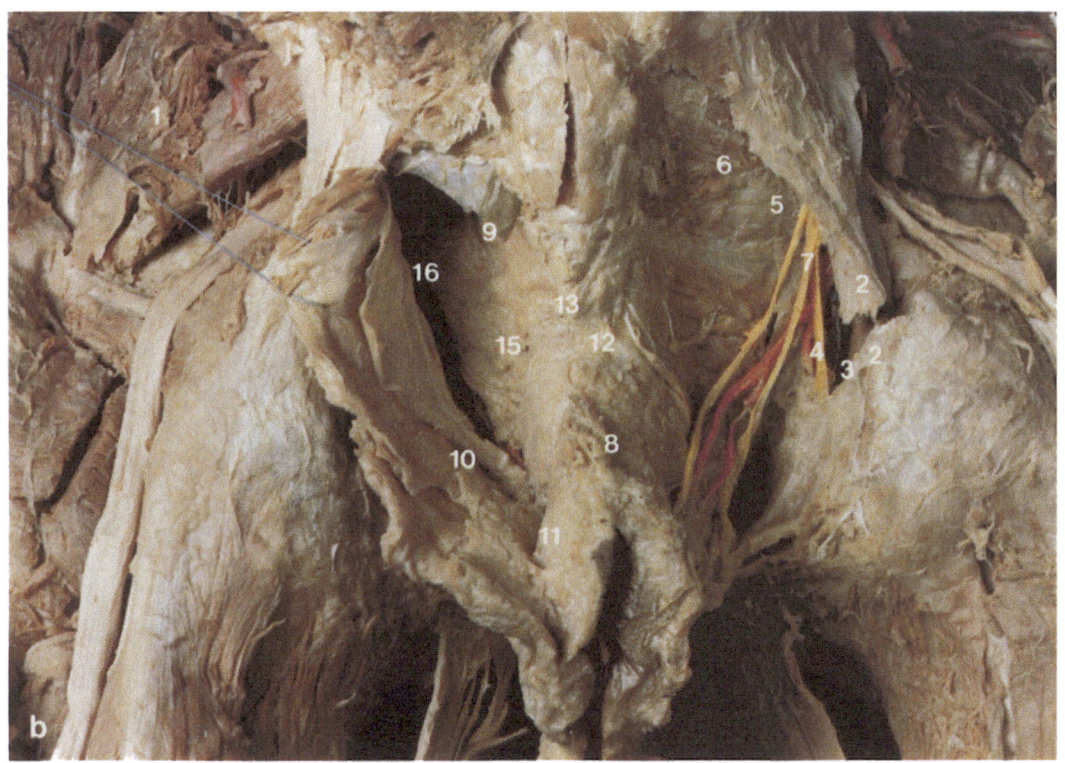

so that the inlet to Alcock's canal (*3*) can be seen. This canal is traversed by the pudendal nerve and pudendal vessels (*4*) after they have left the lesser pelvis and looped around the ischial spine (*5*) and sacrospinous ligament (*6*). The inferior rectal nerves and inferior rectal artery (*7*) which arise in this area have been removed to provide a better view. The sphincters (*8*) are divided in the posterior midline, and the pelvic floor (*9*) is divided by a left parasacral incision. It is apparent that the inner fibers of the levator ani muscle take mainly a longitudinal course in its posterior and distal portions (*10*), becoming blended with the longitudinal muscle coat of the rectum (*11*). Both intraoperatively and in anatomical specimens, one is struck by the variability in the mass and arrangement of the levator ani fibers, and the two telescoping layers that are customarily depicted for this muscle cannot always be distinguished clearly, especially in the elderly. In the present specimen, an internal layer with longitudinal fibers and an external layer with a more circular fiber pattern could be demonstrated, but only through painstaking dissection. In the drawing the union between the levator ani and rectum has been partially dissected. The transverse external fibers of the levator ani merge posteriorally to form the anococcygeal raphe (*12*), which is visible below the resected and anococcygeal ligament (*13*). Distally these external fibers fuse with the deep parts of the external anal sphincter as the puborectalis muscle. Division of the longitudinal muscle coat of the rectum exposes the circular muscle layer, which thickens caudally to form the sphincter ani internus (*14*). The fascial capsule (*15*) of the rectum and the attachments of the lateral fascial wings (the "ailerons lateraux" of French surgeons) (*16*) are visible through the open pelvic floor.

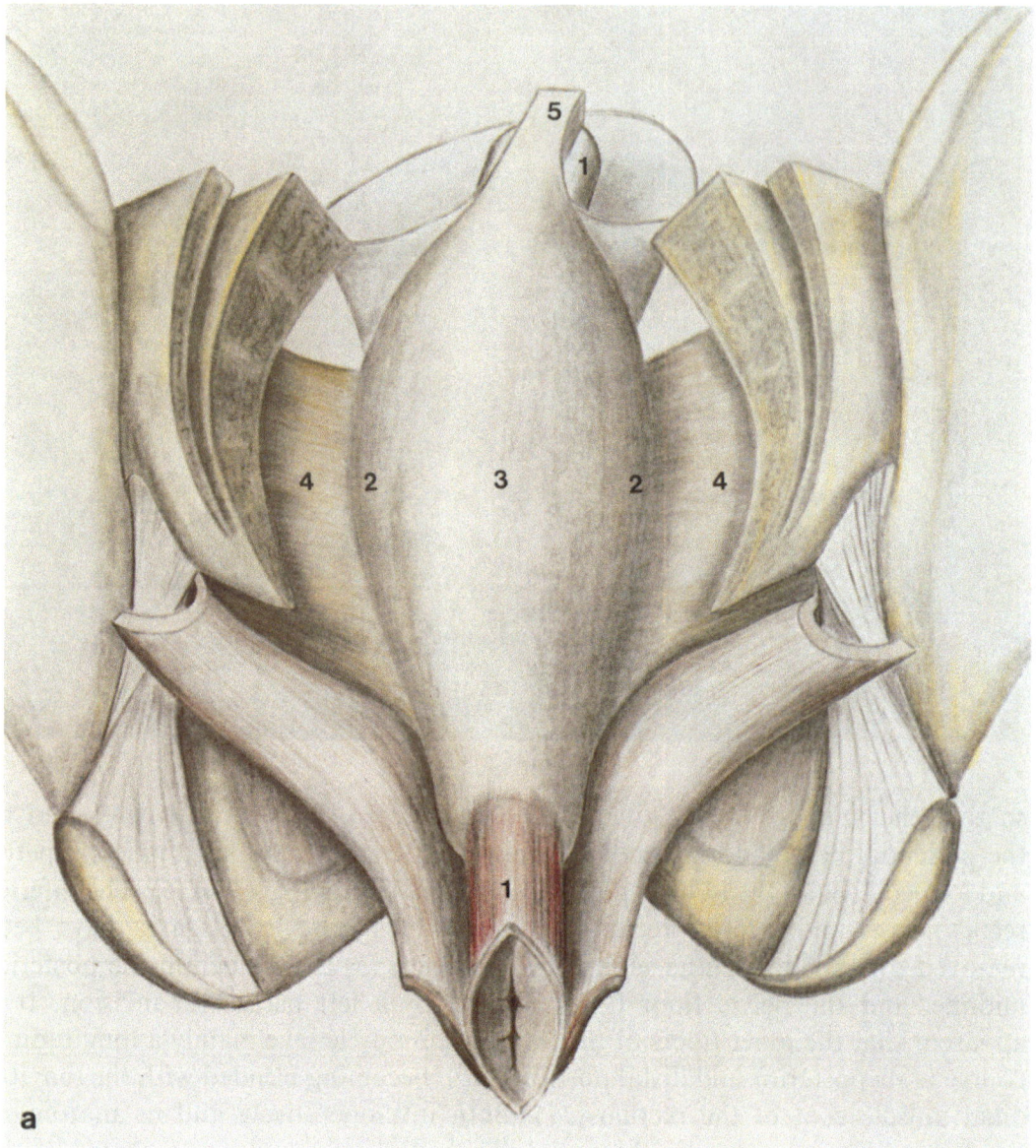

Fig. 4a, b. In the same specimen, the sacrum was sawed in half at the midline to give a broad posterior view of the pelvic interior. The posterior portions of the rectum (*1*) and its fascial capsule (*2*) are well visualized. The term "Waldeyer's fascia" (*3*) actually refers only to the posterior part of the rectal capsule. On each side the fascial capsule is extended to form lateral "wings" (*4*) which are

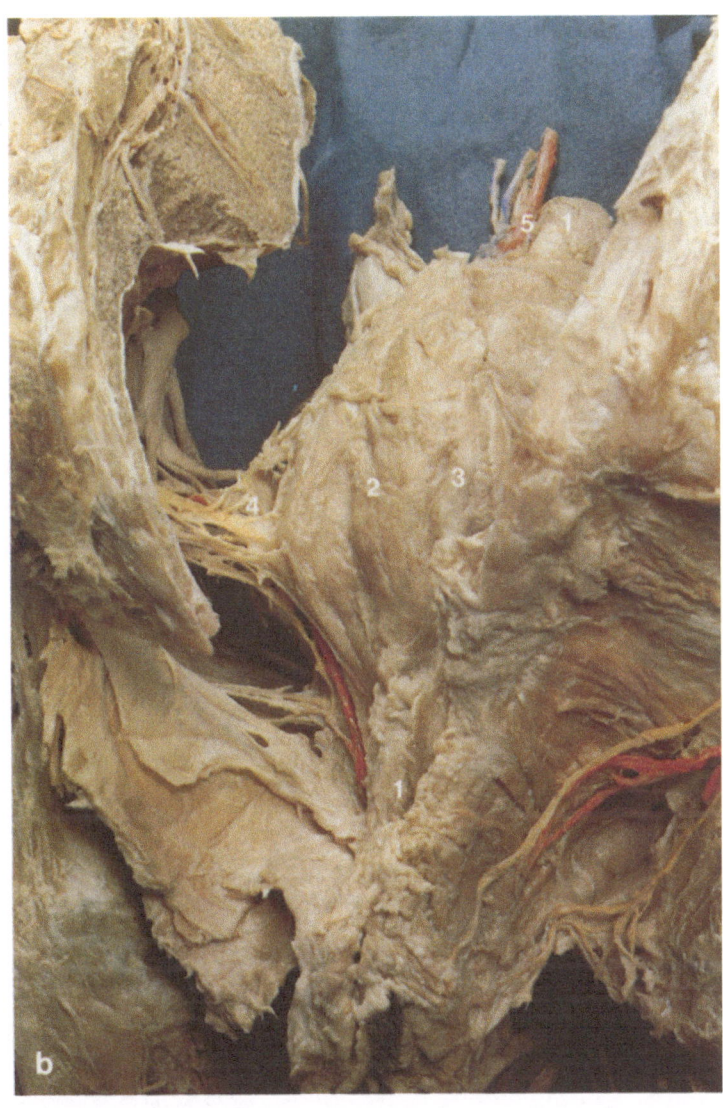

continuous with the pelvic wall, i.e., the internal parietal pelvic fascia. At the junction of the rectum and anal canal, the rectal fascia also is reflected posteriorly onto the parietal pelvic fascia. Cranially, Waldeyer's fascia becomes lost in the connective tissue (5) of the sigmoid mesocolon. Denonvillier's fascia forms the anterior wall of the rectal capsule.

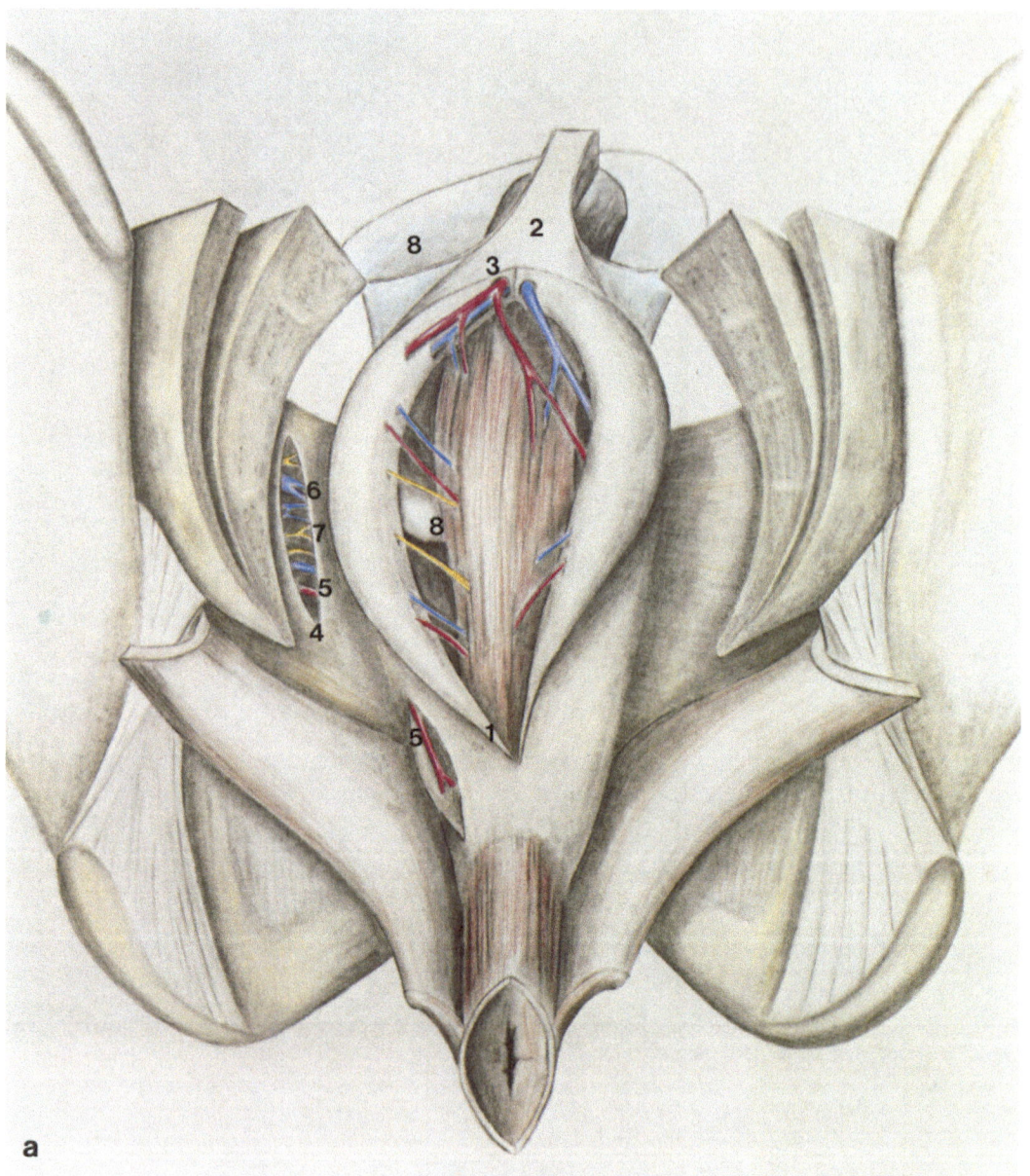

Fig. 5a, b. Waldeyer's fascia is incised longitudinally (*1*) to demonstrate the local nerves and blood vessels supplying the rectum. It will be noted that the nerves and vessels pierce the rectum mainly from the sides, and that few enter from the anterior or posterior aspect.

The superior rectal artery (*3*) descends in the sigmoid mesocolon (*2*) as the terminal branch of the inferior mesenteric artery and enters the fascial capsule of the rectum, accompanied by its veins and the hypogastric nerves. The superior rectal artery usually divides into two branches, occasionally more, which continue to ramify distally and form functional anastomoses with branches of the middle and inferior rectal arteries. Passing through the lateral wings, of which the left

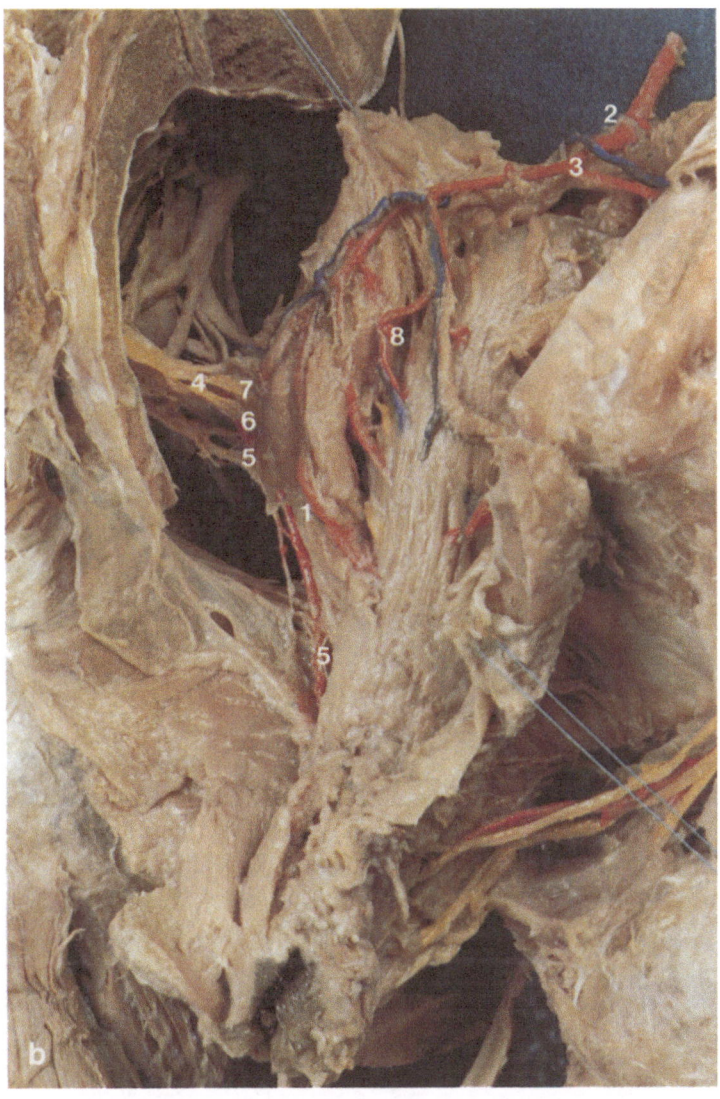

has been cut open (*4*), the middle rectal artery (*5*), venous plexuses (*6*), pelvic splanchnic nerves (nervi erigentes), and communicating branches of the pelvic sympathetic trunk reach the interior of the rectal capsule as autonomic plexuses (*7*). The lateral wings containing the vascular and nerve plexuses have also been termed the mesorecta. Their caudal portions contain few nerves and blood vessels and may be termed the "pars flaccida" of the mesorectum. If the rectum is mobilized for a sufficient distance cranially the rectovesical or rectouterine pouch (of Douglas) (*8*) will be reached.

The peritoneum can be opened at this point, enabling further cranial mobilization of the rectosigmoid.

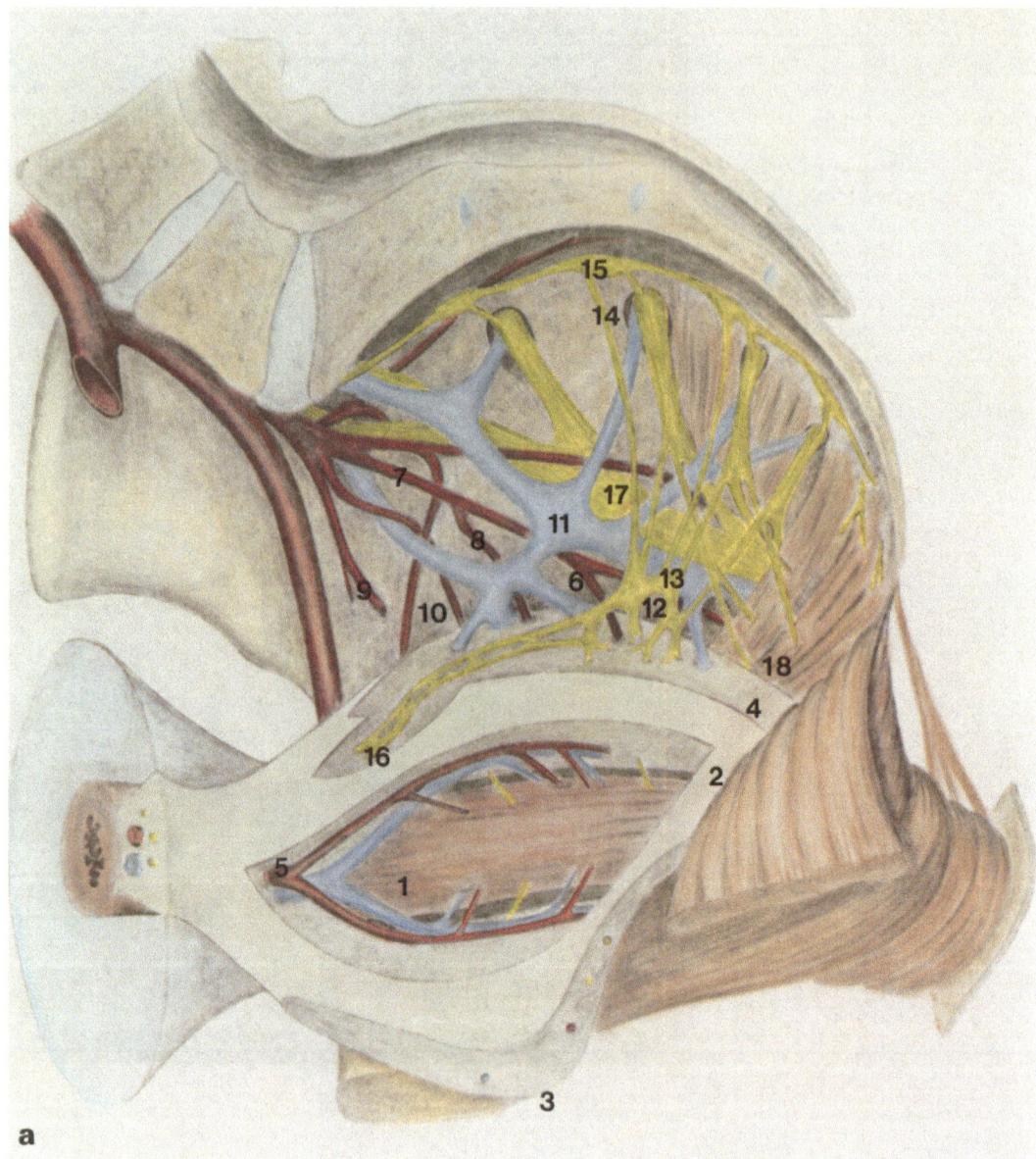

Fig. 6a, b. The model for this drawing is the right half of a male pelvic preparation that has been opened by a left parasagittal incision. The rectum (*1*) and its divided fascial capsule (*2*) have been exteriorized and stretched out. The left lateral wing (*3*) has been divided close to the capsule, and the fascial sheath has been removed from the right wing (*4*). On entering the rectal capsule, the superior rectal artery (*5*) divides into two main branches, which further ramify to anastomose with branches of the middle rectal artery (*6*) and inferior rectal artery. In this specimen the middle rectal artery arises from the internal pudendal (*7*). The artery of the ductus deferens (or uterine artery in the female) (*8*) and the superior (*9*) and inferior vesical arteries (*10*) also traverse the lateral wings to reach their organs of destination. Large venous plexuses (*11*) located in and below the wings drain the organs of the lesser pelvis before emptying into the internal iliac vein. The

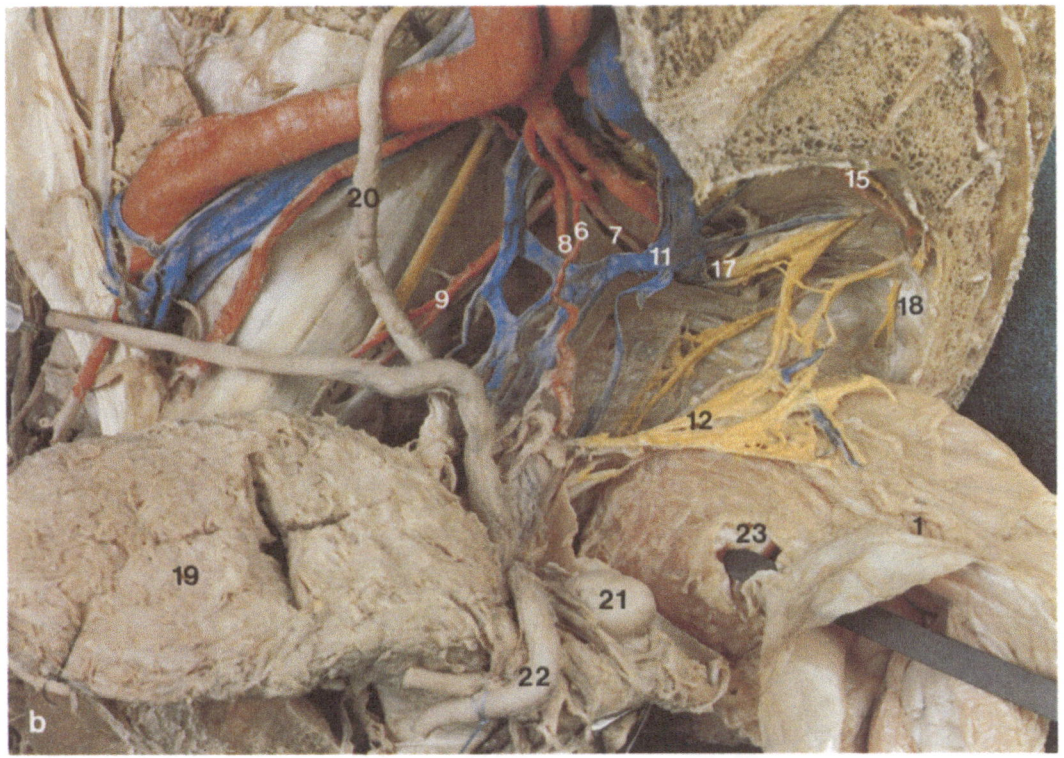

inferior hypogastric plexus (*12*) derives its parasympathetic fibers from the pelvic splanchnic nerves (nervi erigentes) (*13*) of segments S_{2-4}, and its sympathetic fibers from the communicating rami (*14*) of the pelvic sympathetic trunk (*15*) and from the hypogastric nerves (*16*). Like the superior rectal artery, the hypogastric nerves enter the rectal capsule from the superior aspect, establishing connections with the inferior hypogastric plexus. The nerve roots of the sacral segments form the sacral plexus (*17*). Nerve fibers (*18*) arising from $S_{(2)3-4}$ supply the coccygeus and levator ani muscles from the pelvic side. The external sphincters are supplied by nerve fibers which also arise from S_{2-4}, but which follow the course of the pudendal nerve before branching off as the inferior rectal nerves. Urinary bladder (*19*), ureter (*20*), seminal vesicles (*21*), ductus deferens (*22*), rectovesical pouch (*23*).

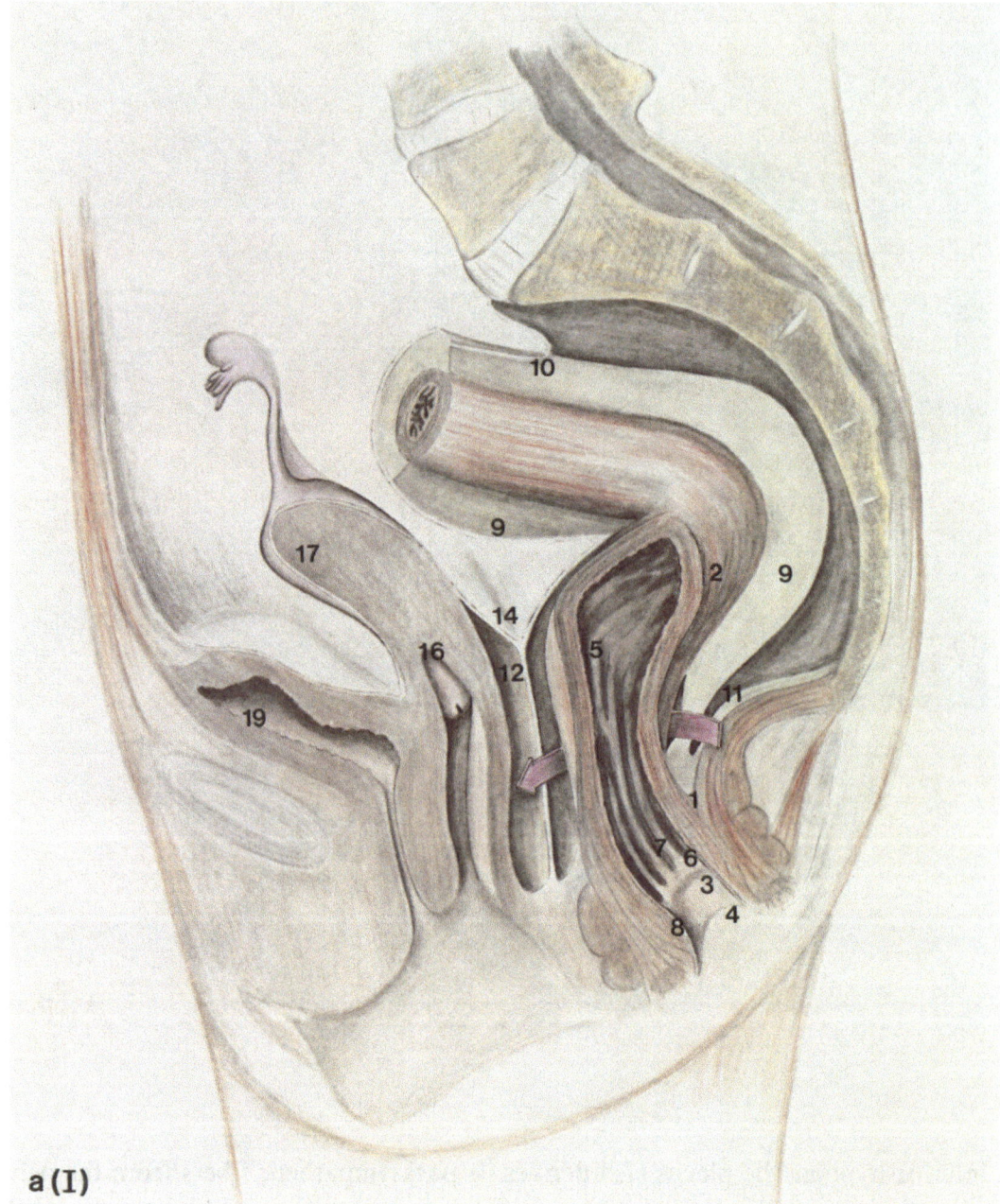

a (I)

Fig. 7a, b (I). The model for this drawing is a female hemipelvis incised in the sagittal plane [cf. male hemipelvis depicted in Fig. 7a, b (II)]. The rectum arises from the sigmoid colon at the point where the free sigmoid mesocolon terminates, or about at the level of the third sacral vertebra. The approximately 15-cm-long segment of rectum located above the rectal diaphragm (1) is known as the pars pelvina (2) or as the rectal ampulla when dilated. Below the rectal diaphragm is the pars perinealis of the rectum (3), which terminates at the anus (4). This subdivision is justified on ontogenic grounds, among others, since the pars pelvina

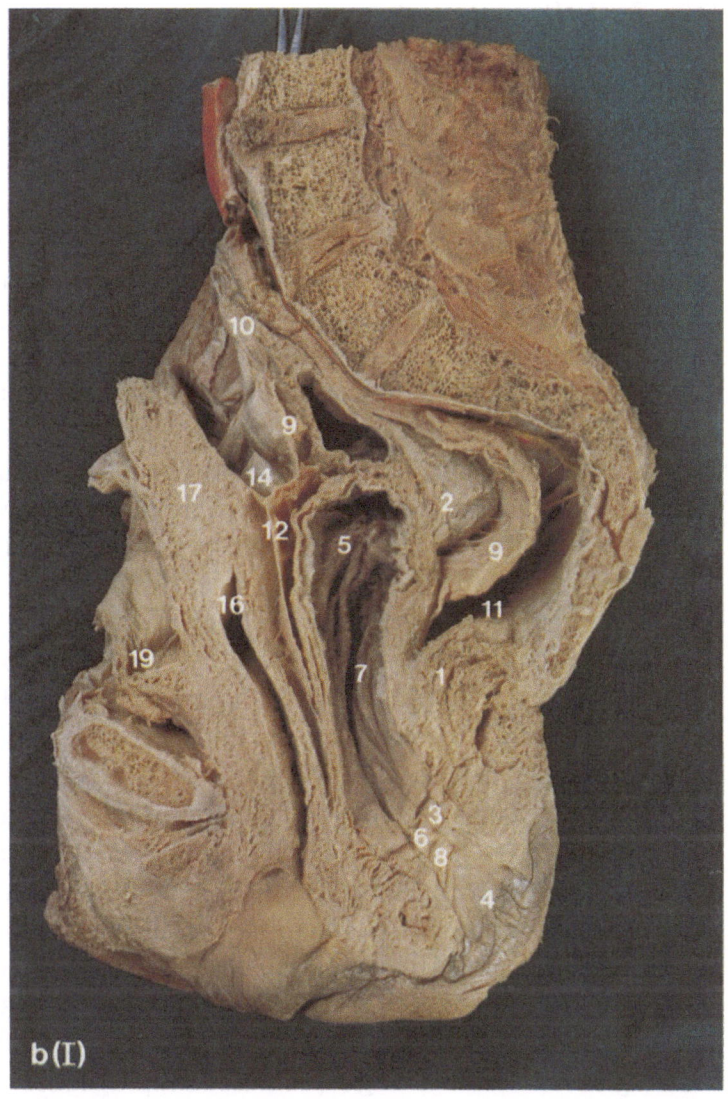

b(I)

develops from the embryonic gut while the pars perinealis is derived from the cloaca.

The cranial half of the pars pelvina is intra-abdominal and retroperitoneal in location, while the caudal half is situated completely outside the abdominal cavity. The pars pelvina describes multiple curves: In the sagittal plane, the sacral flexure is produced as the rectum follows the concavity of the sacrum, and the perineal flexure is produced by the pull of the levator sling. The "anorectal angle" of the perineal flexure measures about 90°. In the frontal plane, the rectum typically curves first to the right and then to the left as it descends. These curves produce infoldings of the mucosa known as the transverse folds (of Houston) (5).

Fig. 7a, b (I) (continued)

Three transverse folds can be distinguished: an upper and a lower fold which protrude into the lumen from the left side, and a middle fold which projects from the right wall. The last-named, known also as Kohlrausch's fold, is situated at the level of the peritoneal reflection (5). In the drawing the uppermost fold is hidden from view by the closed rectum, and the lowest fold has been cut away with the left half. The pars perinealis of the rectum (3) is an alternate name for the anal canal; it commences below the pelvic diaphragm. At the upper border of the approximately 4-cm-long canal is the pectinate line (6). Cords of muscle tissue, blood vessels and lymphatic channels at the end of the pars pelvina create permanent vertical folds in the mucosa called the anal columns (of Morgagni) (7). The recesses between the columns are known as the anal sinuses or crypts, into which the proctodeal glands open. The distal edges of the anal columns and sinuses form a circular, lobed margin (anal valves or pectinate line). The anocutaneous line (of Hilton) (8) marks the lowermost edge of the anal canal.

The pars pelvina of the rectum is enclosed within a fascial capsule (9). The posterior surface of this capsule is known as Waldeyer's fascia. At the sides, the capsule is attached to the pelvic wall by two fascial expansions called the lateral wings, which are continuous with the internal parietal pelvic fascia. These wings are traversed by the blood vessels and nerve plexuses which supply the organs of the lesser pelvis. Cranially, Waldeyer's fascia becomes lost in the retroperitoneal connective tissue of the sigmoid mesocolon (10); distally it is reflected onto the parietal pelvic fascia (11). In the female the anterior surface of the fascial capsule is formed by the rectovaginal fascia (12), and in the male by the prostatoperineal fascia of Denonvillier (13). In embryonic life the peritoneal pocket extends down to the pelvic floor in front of the rectum. As the deep portions of this serosal pouch become obliterated through adhesion, the frontal fascial sheet of Denonvillier is formed. There are occasional reports in the literature that this fascia is lacking in the female, being represented only by loose connective tissue. However, we have found a thick fascial sheet in several female preparations. All that remains of the original serosal pocket extending to the pelvic floor is the rectouterine pouch (14) or rectovesical pouch (15). In this deep portion of the peritoneal sac, the peritoneum in the female is reflected onto the uterus (17) behind the posterosuperior part of the vaginal fornix (16), and in the male onto the urinary bladder (19) level with the upper part of the seminal vesicles (18).

In the present specimen the anorectal angulation was increased when the rectum was mobilized anteriorly out of the sacral cavity. The *arrows* mark the simplest route for obtaining full mobilization of the rectum (cf. Part III).

Fig. 7a, b (II) (see pp. 28/29). This drawing is of a male hemipelvis opened by means of a slightly parasagittal incision [cf. female hemipelvis in *Fig. 7a, b (I)*]. The rectum arises from the sigmoid colon at the point where the free sigmoid mesocolon terminates, or about at the level of the third sacral vertebra. The approximately 15-cm-long segment of rectum located above the rectal diaphragm (*1*) is known as the pars pelvina (*2*) or as the rectal ampulla when dilated. Below the rectal diaphragm is the pars perinealis of the rectum (*3*), which terminates at the anus (*4*). This subdivision is justified on ontogenic grounds, among others, since the pars pelvina develops from the embryonic gut while the pars perinealis is derived from the cloaca.

The cranial half of the pars pelvina is intra-abdominal and retroperitoneal in location, while the caudal half is situated completely outside the abdominal cavity. The pars pelvina describes multiple curves: in the sagittal plane, the sacral flexure is produced as the rectum follows the concavity of the sacrum, while the perineal flexure is produced by the pull of the levator sling. The "anorectal angle" of the perineal flexure measures about 90°. In the frontal plane, the rectum typically curves first to the right and then to the left as it descends. These curves produce infoldings of the mucosa known as the transverse folds (of Houston) (*5*). Three transverse folds can be distinguished: an upper and a lower fold which bulge into the lumen from the left side, and a middle fold which projects from the right wall of the rectum. The last-named, known also as Kohlrausch's fold, is situated at the level of the peritoneal reflection (*5*). In the drawing the uppermost folds is hidden from view by the closed rectum, and the lowest fold has been cut away with the left half. The pars perinealis of the rectum (*3*) is an alternate name for the anal canal; it commences below the pelvic diaphragm. At the upper border of the approximately 4-cm-long canal is the pectinate line (*6*). Cords of muscle tissue, blood vessels and lymphatic channels at the end of the pars pelvina create permanent vertical folds in the mucosa, called the anal columns (of Morgagni) (*7*). The recesses between the columns are known as the anal sinuses or crypts, into which the proctodeal glands open. The distal edges of the anal columns and sinuses form a circular, lobed margin (anal valves or pectinate line). The anocutaneous line (of Hilton) (*8*) marks the lowermost edge of the anal canal.

The pars pelvina of the rectum is enclosed within a fascial capsule (*9*). The posterior surface of this capsule is known as Waldeyer's fascia. At its sides, the capsule is attached to the pelvic wall by two fascial expansions called the lateral wings, which are continuous with the internal parietal pelvic fascia. These wings are traversed by the blood vessels and plexuses which supply the organs of the lesser pelvis. Cranially, Waldeyer's fascia becomes lost in the retroperitoneal connective tissue of the sigmoid mesocolon (*10*); caudally it is reflected onto the parietal pelvic fascia (*11*). The anterior surface of the fascial capsule is formed by the rectovaginal fascia (*12*) in the female and by the prostatoperineal fascia of Denonvillier (*13*) in the male.

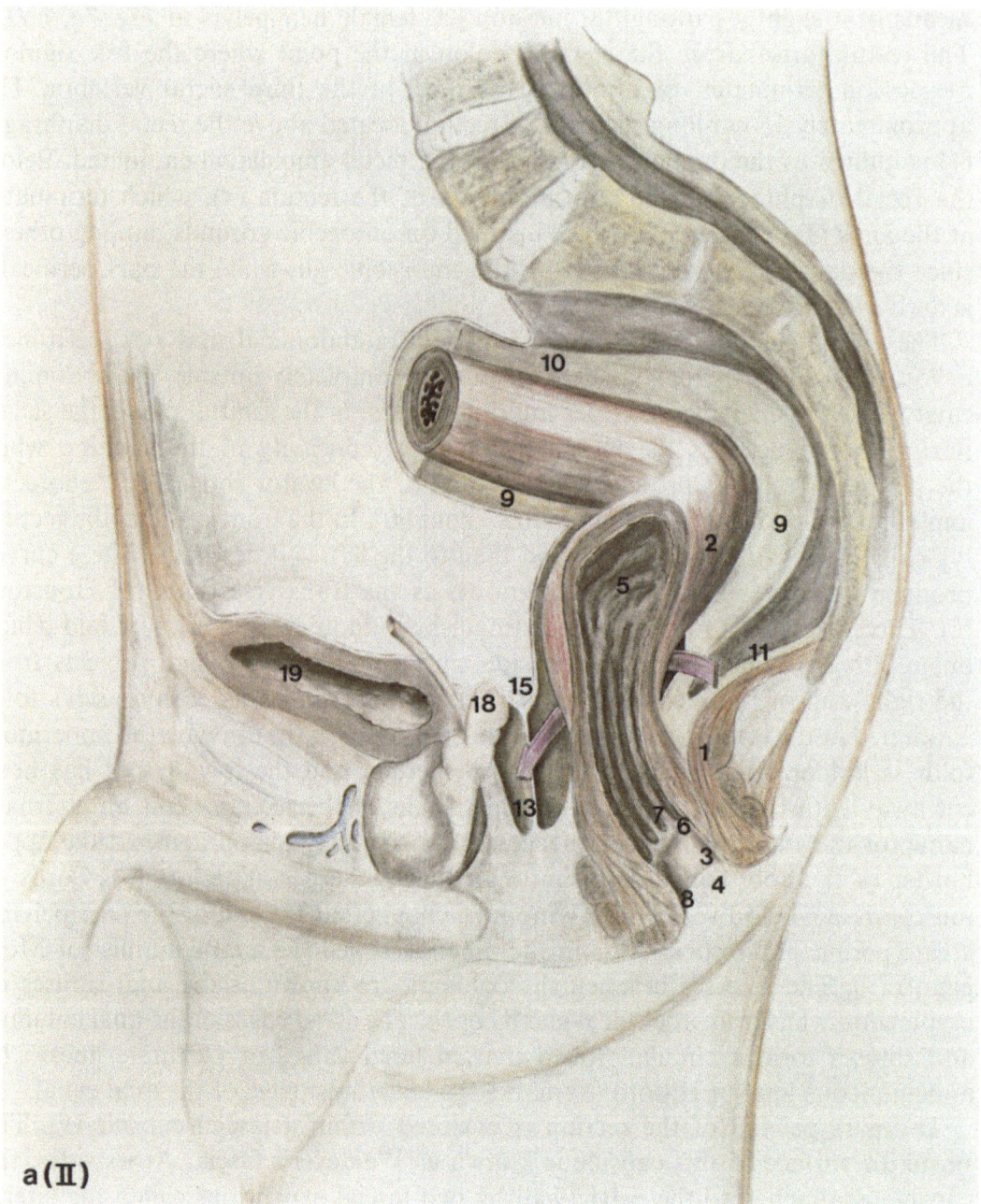

a (II)

Fig. 7a, b (II) *(continued)*
In embryonic life the peritoneal pocket extends down to the pelvic floor in front
of the rectum. As the deep portions of this serosal pouch become obliterated
through adhesion, the frontal fascial sheet of Denonvillier is formed. There are
occasional reports in the literature that this fascia is lacking in the female, being
represented only by loose connective tissue. However, we have found a thick
fascial sheet in several female preparations. All that remains of the original serosal
pocket extending to the pelvic floor is the rectouterine pouch (*14*) or rectovesical

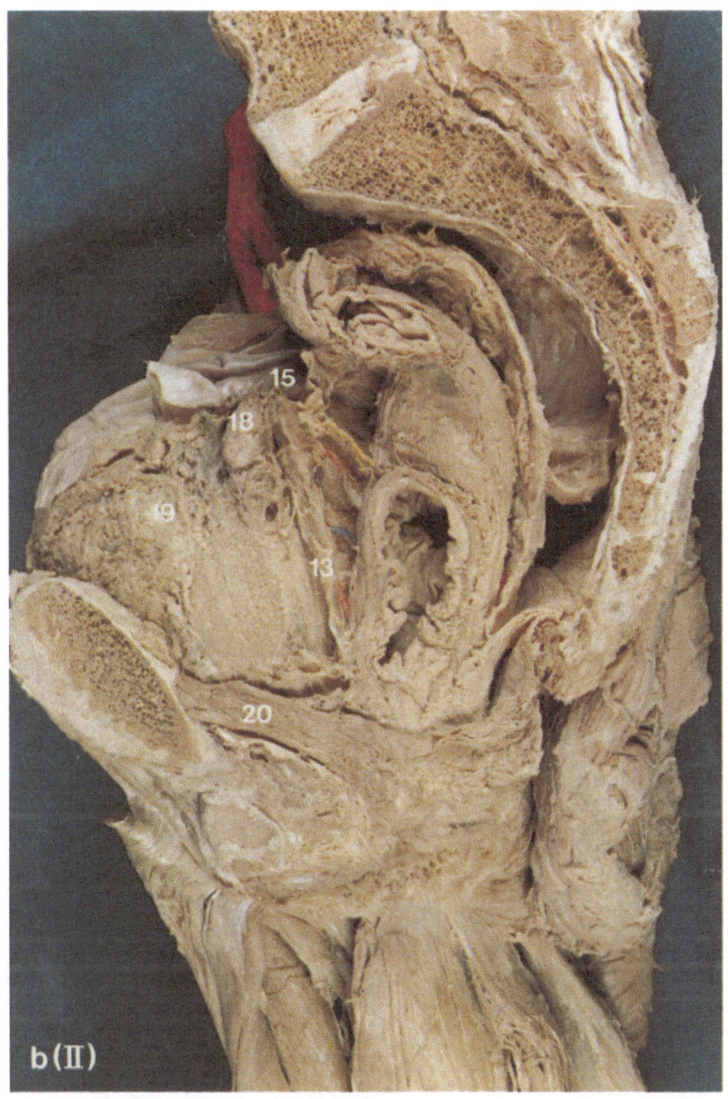

b(II)

pouch (*15*). In this deep portion of the peritoneal sac, the peritoneum in the female is reflected onto the uterus (*17*) behind the posterosuperior part of the vaginal fornix (*16*), and in the male onto the urinary bladder (*19*) level with the upper part of the seminal vesicles (*18*).

In the present specimen, the anorectal anglulation was increased when the rectum was mobilized anteriorly out of the sacral cavity. The *arrows* mark the simplest route for obtaining full mobilization of the rectum (cf. Part III). Note the puborectalis sling (*20*).

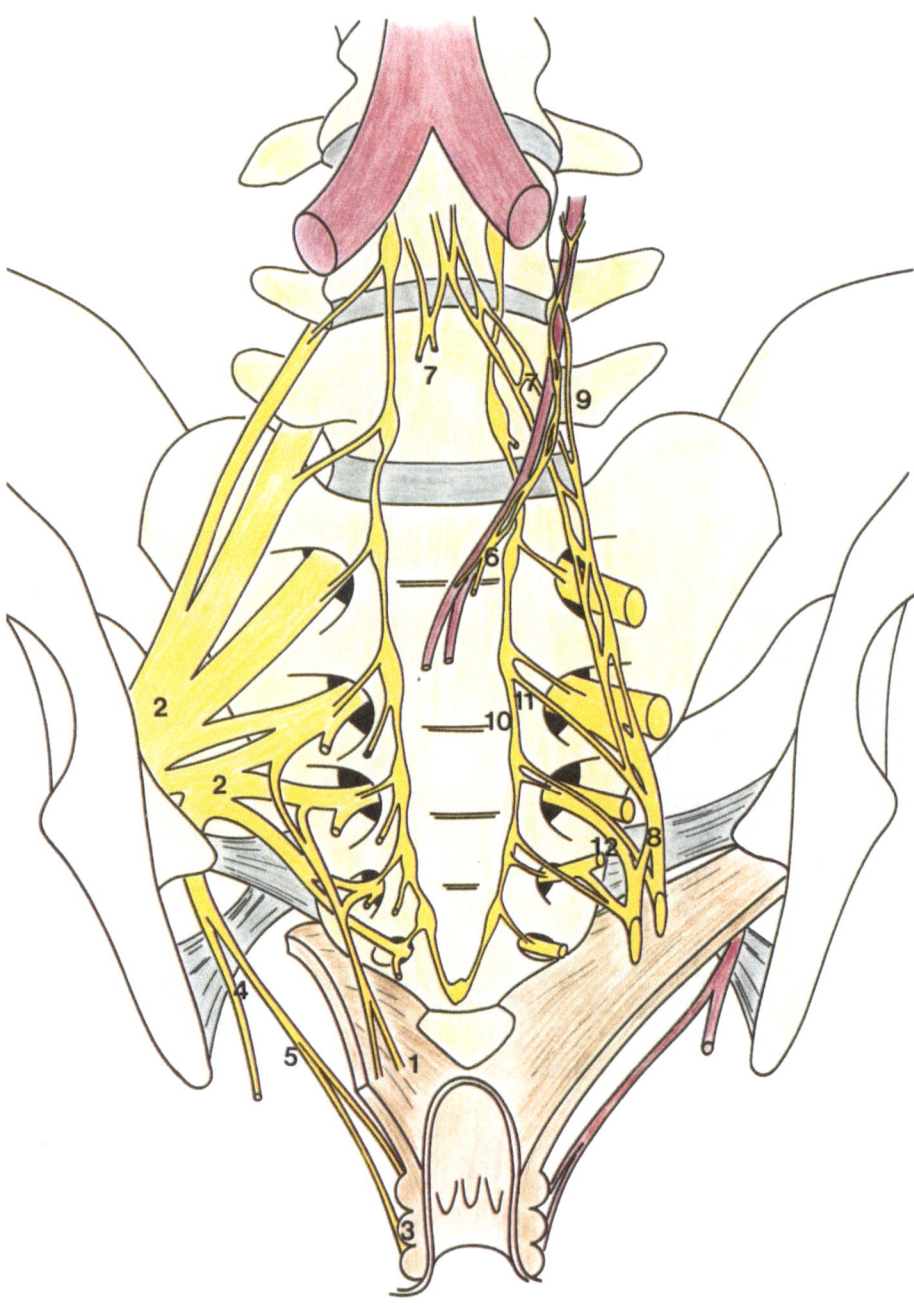

Fig. 8. *Nerve supply*

Levator Ani and Coccygeus. The levator ani (*1*) and coccygeus muscles are supplied with nerve branches from the sacral plexus (*2*). These branches arise from S_3 and S_4 (occasionally from S_{2-4}) and take a posterior-to-anterior course, passing close to the cranial and lateral muscle origins. The nerves generally run along the inner, cranial surface of the muscles, but individual fibers occasionally pierce the levator ani muscle and course a short distance on its inferior surface before passing back through the muscle to its inner surface.

In some cases the levator ani is supplied by an accessory nerve which arises from the same sacral segments, but which courses on the outer surface of the muscle sheet.

Puborectalis. The puborectalis muscle derives its nerve supply from S_{2-4}. Reports vary as to whether the nerve branches supplying the puborectalis arise from the pudendal nerve or directly from the sacral nerve roots, i.e., whether they course on the outer surface of levator ani or on its inner, pelvic surface. Shepherd (1980) describes a pudendal innervation of the puborectalis, while Percy et al. (1981) found that the puborectalis sling was supplied by pelvic branches from $S_{3,4}$. Ontogenically the puborectalis, like the external sphincters, is derived from the cloacal sphincter muscle, which is supplied by the pudendal nerve. Lawson (1981), drawing on the work of Uhlenhuth (1953), Holl (1897) and Gorsch (1941), divides the muscle into a cranial part and a caudal part, with the cranial part supplied by pelvic nerves and the caudal part by branches of the pudendal. We cannot furnish a definitive answer to this question based on our work on anatomical preparations. We have found variable ascending and descending nerve branches at the junction of the puborectalis and external sphincter.

Sphincter Ani Externus. The sphincter ani externus (*3*) is supplied by branches from the pudendal nerve (*4*). The corresponding fibers arise from S_{2-4} (the sacral plexus). The branches to the sphincter ani externus leave Alcock's canal to reach their muscles as the inferior rectal nerves (*5*).

Sphincter Ani Internus. Being a smooth, visceral muscle, the sphincter ani internus derives its nerve supply from the inferior hypogastric plexus. It should be stressed that there are no intramural ganglia of Auerbach's plexus in the sphincter ani internus, and that the question of whether cholinergic nerves have an excitatory action and adrenergic nerves have an inhibitory action, or vice-versa, has not yet been resolved.

Rectum. The rectum derives its innervation from both the sympathetic and para-sympathetic systems and from afferent pathways. The nerve fibers reach the rectum via the superior rectal plexus and inferior hypogastric plexus.

Sympathetic Nerve Supply. The sympathetic fibers to the rectum are derived from the first two lumbar segments of the spinal cord. From the upper lumbar ganglia of the sympathetic trunk, the fibers pass to the abdominal aortic plexus. From there some pass to the rectum via the inferior mesenteric plexus (*6*), accompanied by the artery of the same name. Others pass through the superior hypogastric plexus (hypogastric nerves) (*7*) to the inferior hypogastric (pelvic) plexus (*8*) before reaching the rectum. The hypogastric nerves also receive fibers (*9*) from the inferior mesenteric plexus.

Fibers (*11*) from the sacral ganglia of the sympathetic trunk (*10*) radiate into the inferior hypogastric plexus and supply the rectum.

Fig. 8 (continued)

At present it is believed that the most important sympathetic pathway to the pelvis and rectum is that which passes through the inferior hypogastric plexus. Modern theory holds that the sympathetic nerves of the rectum are devoid of afferent fibers. A sympathectomy of the rectum, in any case, has no obvious physiological effects.

Parasympathetic Nerve Supply. The 2nd, 3rd and 4th segments of the sacral parasympathetic center supply the rectum. The parasympathetic fibers branch off from the corresponding sacral nerves as the pelvic splanchnic (nervi erigentes) (*12*), which enter the inferior hypogastric plexus and from there pass to the rectum. A portion of the fibers ascend from the inferior hypogastric plexus via the hypogastric nerves to enter the inferior mesenteric plexus, from which they are distributed to the sigmoid colon and descending colon. The sacral parasympathetic fibers are followed in their course by the visceral afferent fibers.

Visceral Afferent Fibers. The rectum and anal canal are both supplied by afferent fibers from S_{2-4}.

The visceral afferent fibers of the rectum and upper anal canal arise from the sacral nerves just outside the sacral foramina and pass with the parasympathetic fibers in the pelvic splanchnic (nervi erigentes) to the inferior hypogastric plexus. From here they supply the anorectum as far cranially as the rectosigmoid junction and as far caudally as the pectinate line.

The visceral afferent fibers of the anal canal and the afferent fibers of the perineal skin course within the pudendal nerve before branching off as the inferior rectal nerves, accompanied by the voluntary motor fibers of the external sphincter. These inferior rectal branches course along the lower surface of the levator ani muscle to reach the lower anal canal and perineal skin.

The skin of the anal canal, like that of the body in general, is sensitive to touch, heat, cold and pain. The rectal mucosa, on the other hand, lacks sensation. The boundary of sensation, i.e. of somatic and visceral afferent innervation, is situated at the pectinate line or about 1 cm above it. As in the remainder of the bowel, wall tension and ischemia can produce pain in the rectum. But while the pain fibers in the rest of the bowel are a part of the sympathetic system, those of the rectum follow parasympathetic pathways. It appears, in fact, that all afferent fibers of the rectum belong to the parasympathetic system.

Muscular Afferent Fibers. Various authors have reported finding stretch receptors in the sphincter ani externus and levator ani muscles (Winckler 1958; Walls 1959). The interaction of these receptors with the visceral afferent fibers, reflex arcs, and the motor nerve supply of the external sphincter and levator are responsible for neuromuscular continence. It should be remembered, however, that the pars pelvina of the rectum with its visceral afferent fibers can be completely resected without causing significant disturbances of defecation and continence. It may be concluded, then, that the pars pelvina and particularly its visceral afferent fibers are not essential for defecation and continence. As mentioned earlier, the puborectalis muscle appears to play a crucial role in maintaining continence. Even in the absence of a normal anal canal, rectum and internal and external sphincter, the sensory and motor capabilities of an intact puborectalis sling are sufficient to provide an acceptable degree of continence in conjunction with the reservoir function of the neorectum.

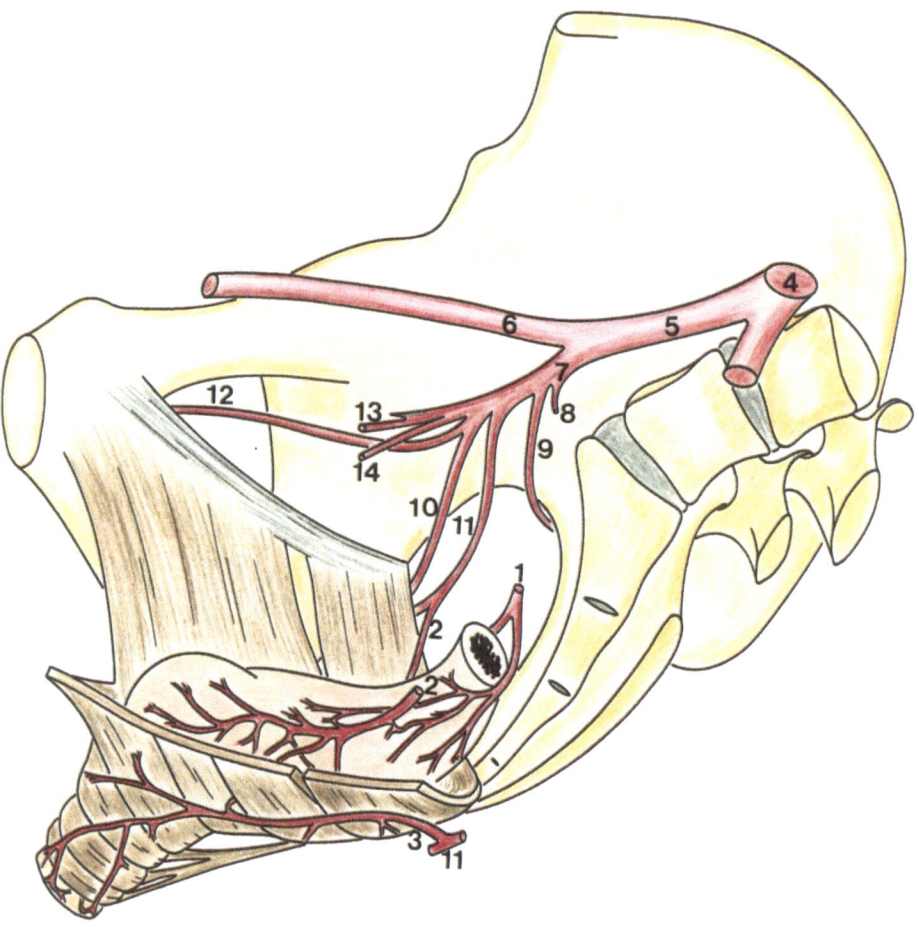

Fig. 9. *Blood supply.* Blood is supplied to the rectum at three levels, all of which interconnect through functional anastomoses. The upper level is formed by the unpaired superior rectal artery, a large terminal branch of the inferior mesenteric. At the middle level, the rectum is supplied by the left and right middle rectal arteries. At the lower level, the inferior rectal artery supplies the rectum, the anal region, the external sphincters, and the levator ani.

1 Superior rectal artery
2 Middle rectal artery
3 Inferior rectal artery
4 Aorta
5 Common iliac artery
5 External iliac artery
7 Internal iliac artery
8 Lateral sacral artery

9 Superior gluteal artery
10 Inferior gluteal artery
11 Internal pudendal artery
12 Obturator artery
13 Superior vesical artery
    with lateral umbilical lig.
14 Inferior vesical artery

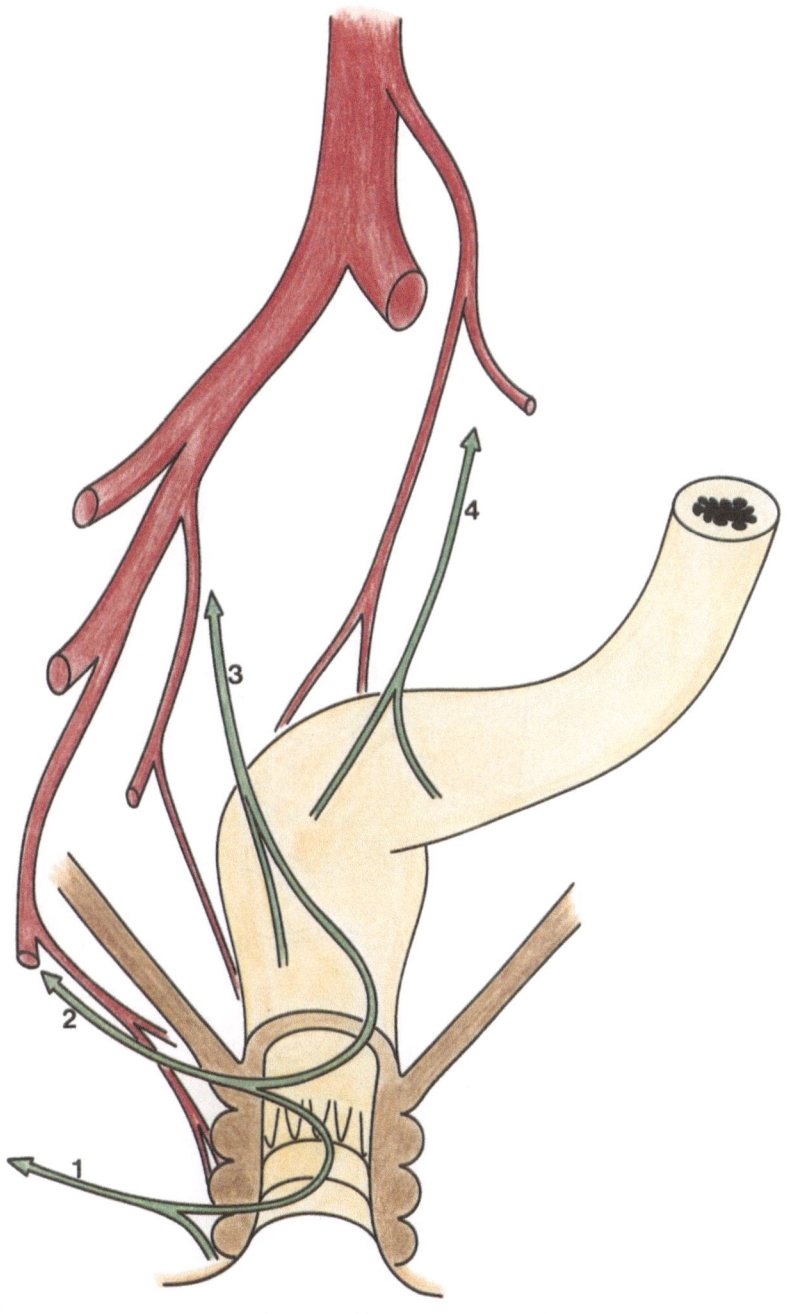

Fig. 10. *Lymphatic drainage.* The lymphatic vessels of the rectum form an expansive, coherent network. Lymph from the region of the anus drains to the inguinal lymph nodes. Lymph drainage from the pars perinealis of the anal canal occurs mainly along the inferior rectal and pudendal vessels, while lymph from the lower portion of the pars pelvina drains mainly along the middle rectal vessels to the internal iliac nodes. Lymph from the upper parts of the rectum drains along the superior rectal vessels to the para-aortic lymph nodes. Inguinal nodes (*1*), internal iliac nodes (*2, 3*), para-aortic nodes (*4*).

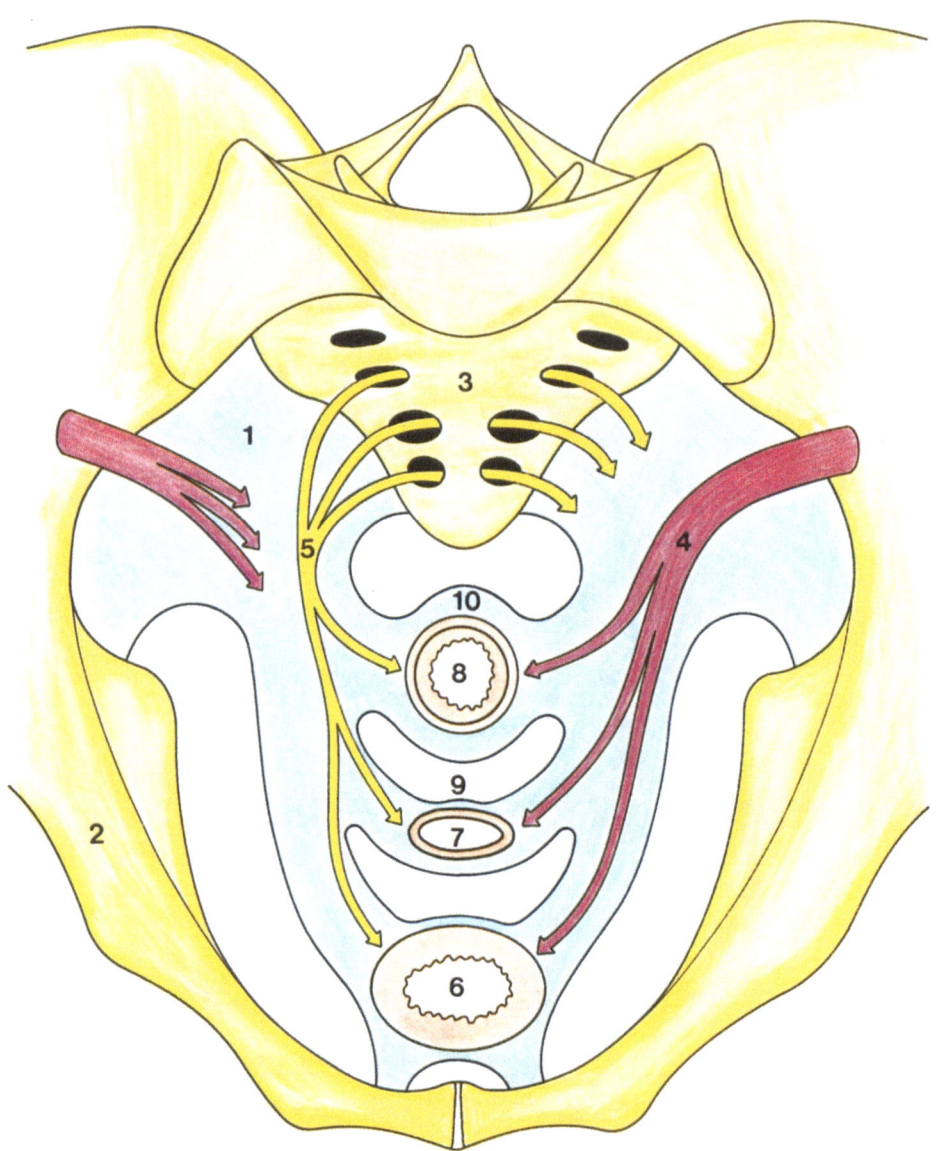

Fig. 11. *Lateral wing, axial view.* The large vascular trunks and nerve pathways of the pelvic organs pass through the lateral fascial wings of the rectum. Through a posterior incision in Waldeyer's fascia, circumferential mobilization of the rectum can be carried out with ease and safety.

1 Lateral wing
2 Pelvic ring
3 Sacrum
4 Blood vessels of the pelvic organs
5 Parasympathetic nerve pathways
  of the pelvic organs

6 Bladder
7 Uterus
8 Rectum
9 Pouch of Douglas
10 Waldeyer's fascia

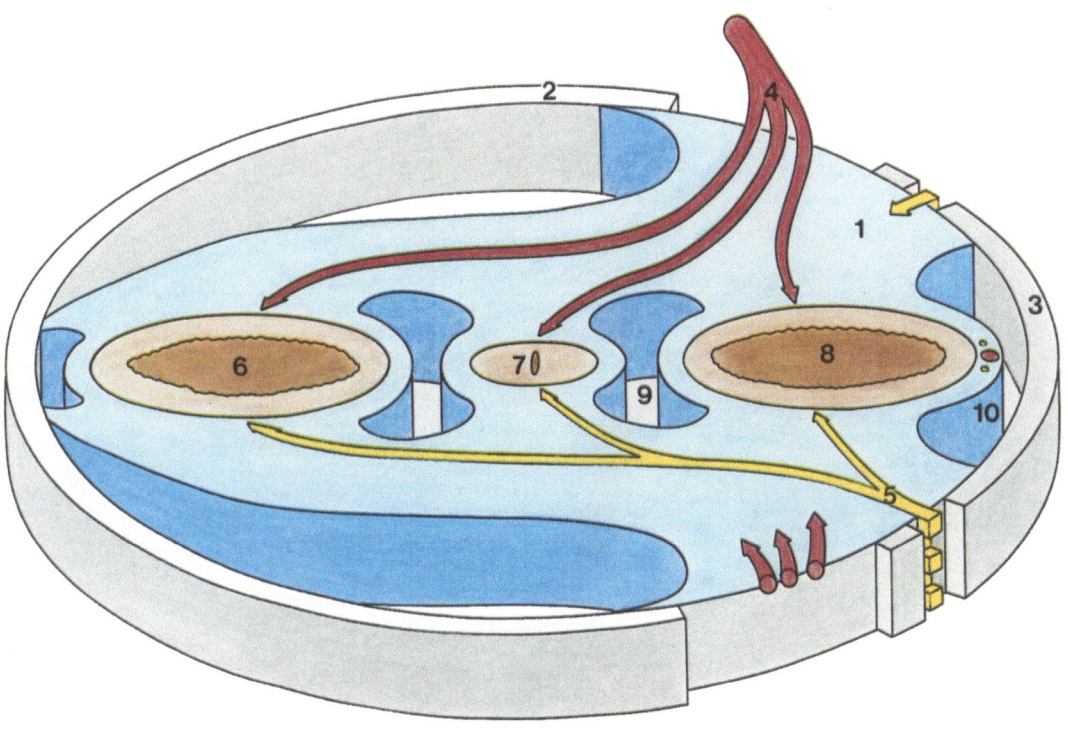

Fig. 12. *Lateral wing, oblique view.* The large vascular trunks and nerve pathways of the pelvic organs pass through the lateral fascial wings of the rectum. Through a posterior incision in Waldeyer's fascia, circumferential mobilization of the rectum can be carried out with ease and safety.

1 Lateral wing
2 Pelvic ring
3 Sacrum
4 Blood vessels of the pelvic organs
5 Parasympathetic nerve pathways
  of the pelvic organs

6 Bladder
7 Uterus
8 Rectum
9 Pouch of Douglas
10 Waldeyer's fascia

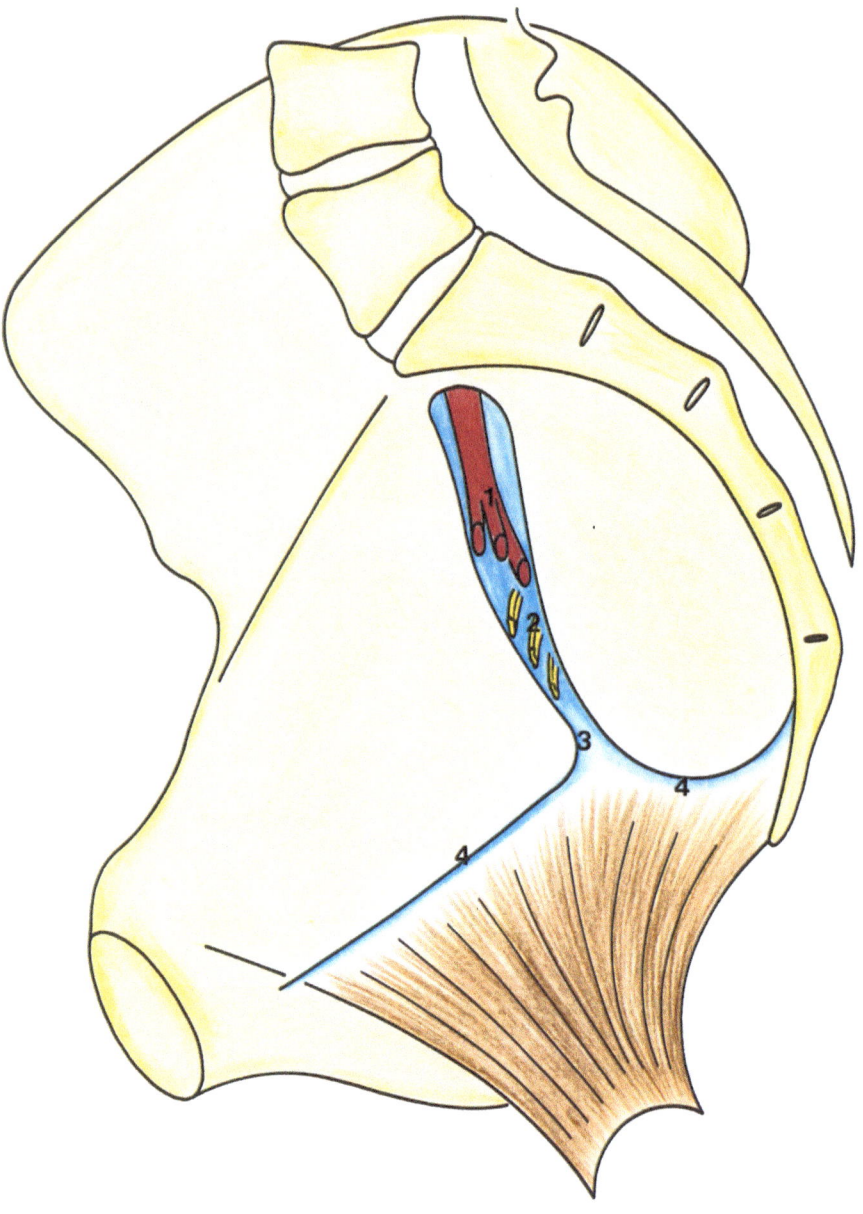

Fig. 13. *Lateral wing, parietal view.*

1 Vascular trunks of the pelvic organs
2 Parasympathetic nerve pathways of the pelvic organs
3 Pars flaccida of the lateral wing
4 Parietal reflection of the lateral wing

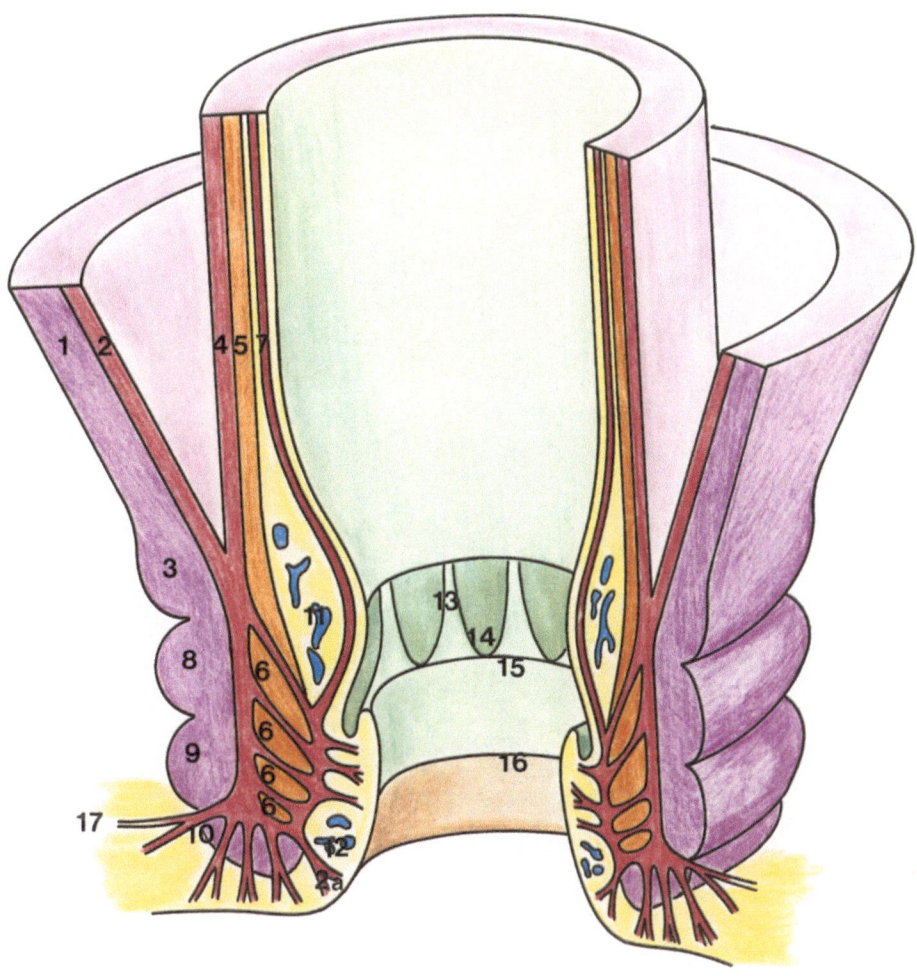

Fig. 14. *Rectum, anus and pelvic floor.* In the region of the anal canal, where the bowel leaves the peritoneal cavity, the rectum is intimately adherent to the body wall, making it difficult to surgically define the various layers. This also prevents isolated mobilization of the rectum in that area. The inner layer of longitudinal levator ani fibers blends with the longitudinal muscle coat of the rectum. It is advantageous to start the incision of the pelvic floor and rectal mobilization above the level of the "rectolevator sinus."

 1 Levator ani, circular layer
 2 Levator ani, longitudinal layer
2a Corrugator ani (extension of the inner layer of levator ani)
 3 Puborectalis
 4 Longitudinal muscle coat of rectum
 5 Circular muscle coat of rectum
 6 Sphincter ani internus (inferior border: pecten band)
 7 Muscularis mucosae

 8 Sphincter ani externus, deep part
 9 Sphincter ani externus, superficial part
10 Sphincter ani externus, subcutaneous part
11 Internal hemorrhoidal plexus
12 External hemorrhoidal plexus
13 Anal columns
14 Anal crypts
15 Pectinate line
16 Anocutaneous line (of Hilton)
17 Transverse septum of the ischiorectal fossa

Part III
Operative Technique

Introduction

In the following, the operative technique of the transsphincteric approach to the rectum is described as it was practised on over 80 patients in the initial phase of study in the Department of Surgery at the Kantonsspital Basel.

Here, it should once again be emphasized how important preparation is to the operation. Thorough orthograde intestinal lavage and a correct Heidelberg position, with carefully performed anesthesia, facilitate the surgical intervention and are essential to favorable postoperative progress.

A precise awareness of topographic anatomy has proven to be extremely helpful and has made possible the further development and refinement of the operative technique. This has been particularly effective in the difficult phase of skeletalization of the rectum and its resection with "perirectal fat."

Opinion is divided as to whether a primary protective colostomy should be established. In our experience, such a procedure is superfluous when the operation is performed on an empty and well-lavaged rectum and the anastomosis has been satifactorily carried out.

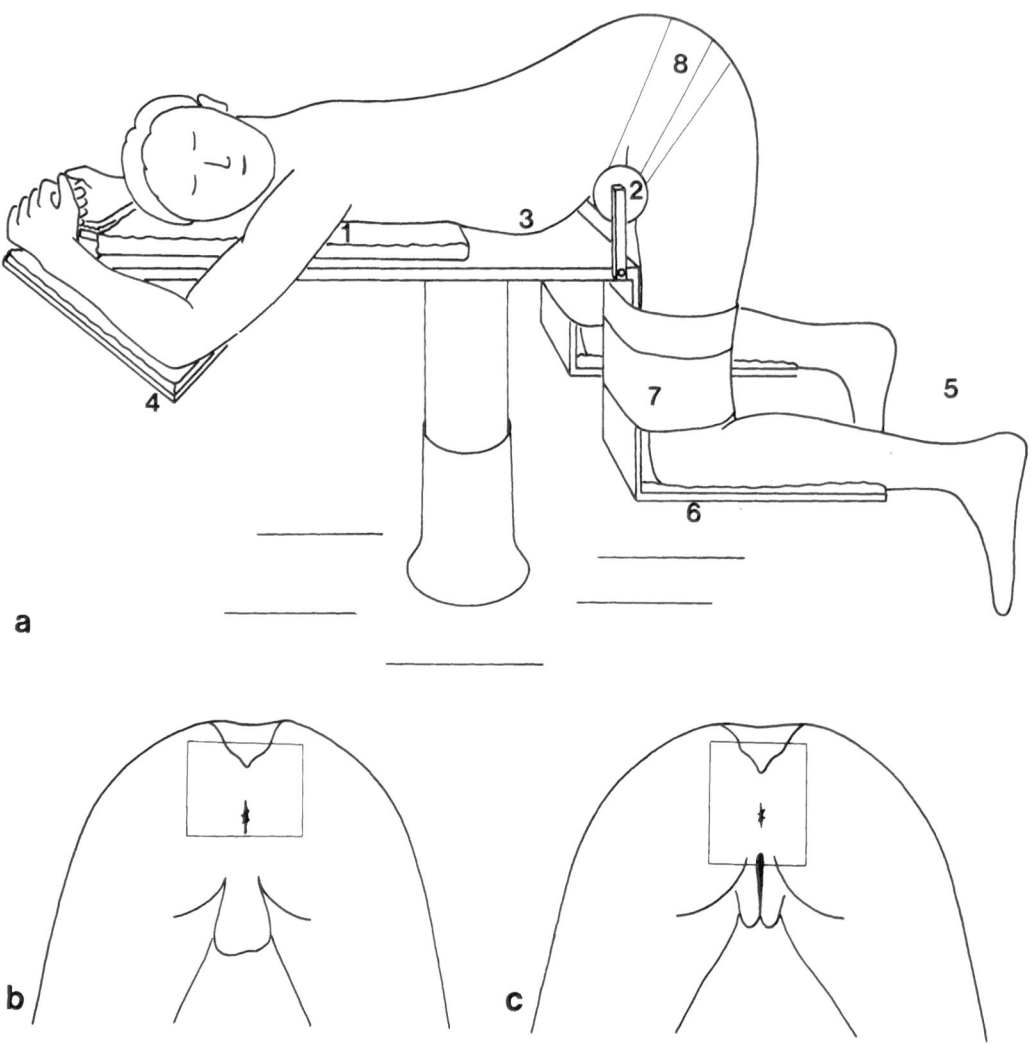

Fig. 15a–c. a Patient in the Heidelberg position for transsphincteric surgery. Firm foam-rubber cushions (*1*) are placed beneath the chest and the head, which is turned to the side. The pelvic ring is well supported by a foam-rubber roll (*2*), while the abdomen (*3*) is unsupported to allow free respiratory movements. The arms are supported on padded rests (*4*) which are mounted somewhat below table level to reduce abduction and elevation of the arms and thus avoid plexus injury. The legs are well abducted (*5*) so that the operator can work freely between them. The legs are flexed 90° at the hip and knee joints with the knees and lower legs resting on padded splints (*6*) below table level. The thighs are strapped to the table over padding (*7*). The buttocks are taped apart (*8*) to facilitate access to the pelvic floor. The operative area measures approximately 25 × 30 cm. The sacrum, anus and vagina are draped free (**b** and **c**).

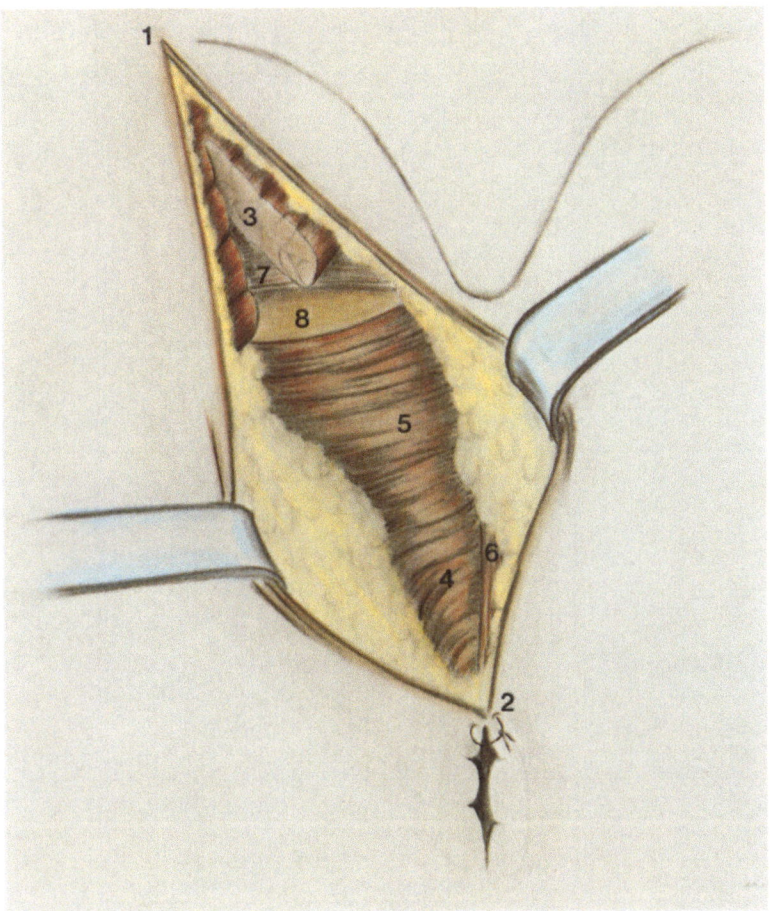

Fig. 16. The left parasacral skin incision (*1*) begins about 3 fingerwidths above the tip of the sacrum and extends obliquely downward, parallel to the sacrum and 1 fingerwidth from it, to the anocutaneous line in the midline, where the endpoint of the incision is marked with a knotted suture. If a complete transsphincteric division of the anal canal is proposed, two knots are placed at this location – one to the left of the incision and one to the right (see Fig. 18). The wound edges are retracted, and the subcutaneous fat is incised. When the border of the gluteus maximus muscle (*3*) comes into view, it is notched to expose the external sphincters (*4*), the levator ani (*5*), the anococcygeal ligament (*6*) and the sacrospinous ligament (*7*). The sphincters are very difficult to identify individually during surgery, as is their junction with the levator ani. The space (*8*) between the levator ani and sacrospinous ligament may gape very widely at this stage.

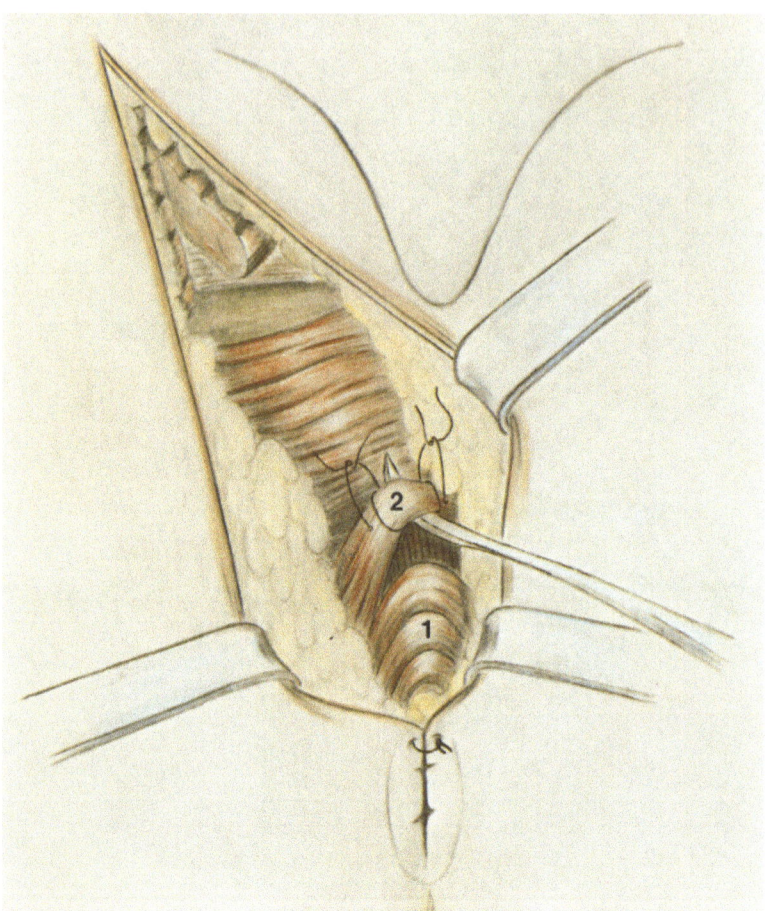

Fig. 17. While the sphincters generally do not have to be divided for the resection of a rectal prolapse, a sphincterotomy is almost always indicated for tumor surgery owing to the superior access that it affords. The external sphincters (*1*) are intimately blended with the pars perinealis of the rectum and cannot be easily separated from it. Thus, dividing these muscles without perforating the bowel requires clear identification of the layers and a meticulous working technique. It is easier to start the division of the levator ani further cranially (*2*), where the muscle is separate from the rectum. The surgeon should keep as close to the midline as possible in order to spare the nerve and blood supply of the sphincters and levator ani. If transsphincteric division of the anal canal is necessary, this may now be done in a cranial-to-caudal fashion. The levator insertion and anococcygeal ligament are detached from the tip of the sacrum ("posterior release"). The muscle layers are then divided between ligatures, whose ends are left long and marked with knots. Failure to mark the muscle layers at the time of division can make later identification and repair extremely difficult (cf. Fig. 19).

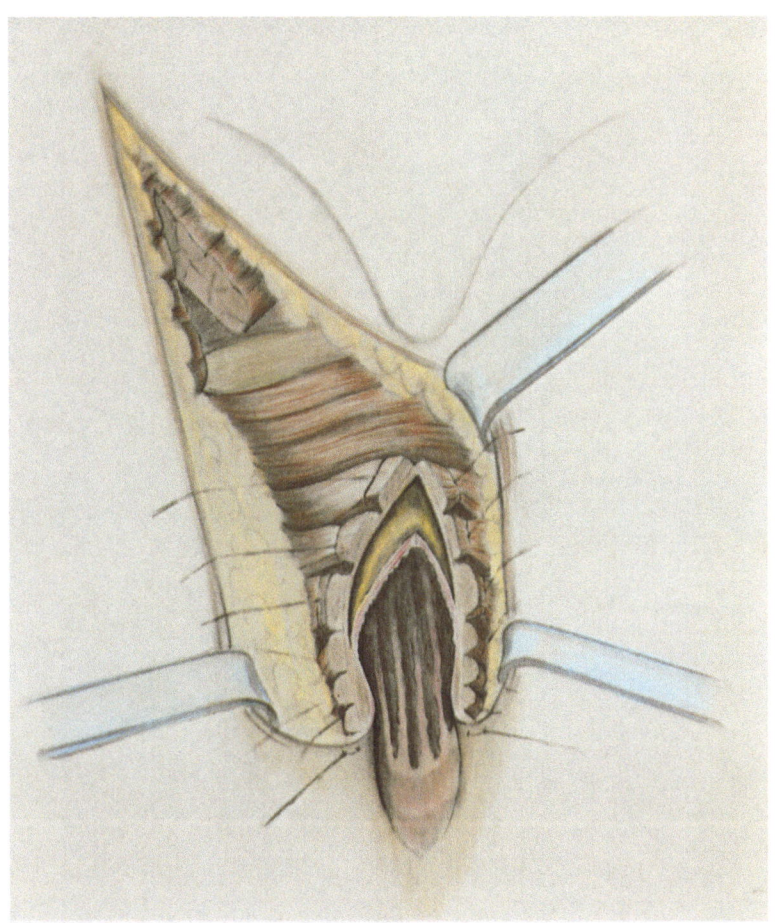

Fig. 18. A longitudinal posterior incision has been made through the sphincters and anal canal. This incision affords excellent exposure of low-sited rectal tumors. For simplicity, the anal canal is not shown incised in the remaining illustrations on surgical technique.

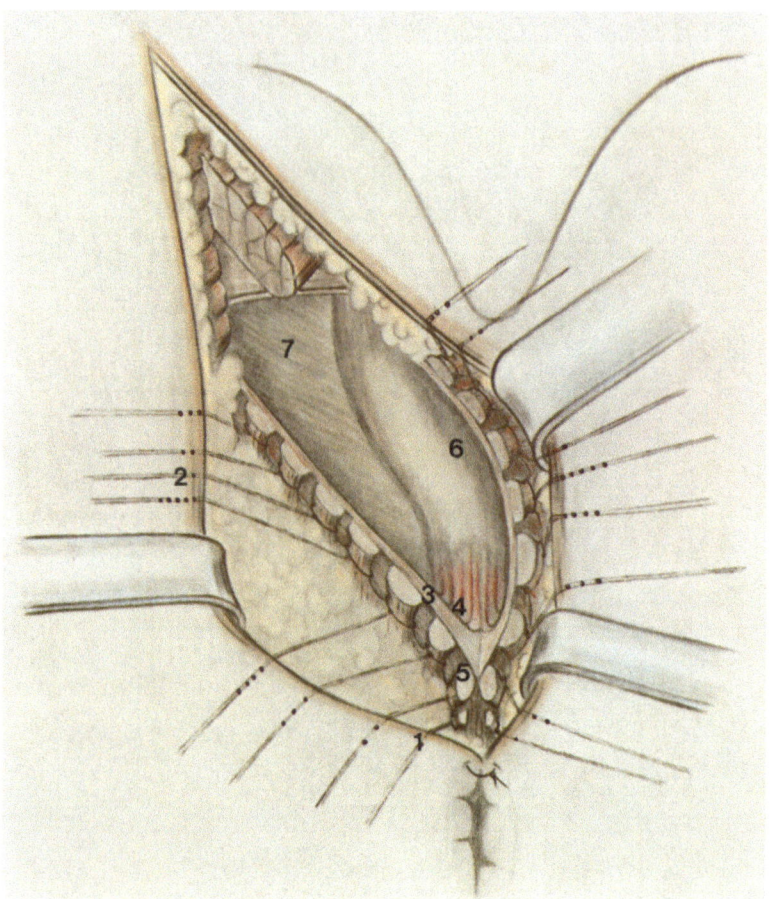

Fig. 19. The levator ani and external sphincters are shown completely divided. The individual muscle layers are lifted on a Kocher probe and divided between paired identifying sutures. For this and all other stages of the operation, we use 3/0 or 2/0 absorbable polyglycol sutures (Dexon), tying equal numbers of knots in each suture pair (*1*) to mark the matching muscle edges. If the number of knots exceeds five, it is best to change the size or colour of the sutures and begin again with one knot (*2*). An operator who is well acquainted with the anatomy of this region may need fewer identifying sutures than one who is not. Note that the inner muscle fibers of the levator ani run longitudinally, and that it and the fascia of the internal pelvic diaphragm are divided longitudinally as one layer (*3*). The surgeon should maintain the integrity of the muscle-fascia sheet to the greatest extent possible, as this will facilitate pelvic floor reconstruction. Note that the inner, longitudinal fibers of levator ani blend with the longitudinal muscle coat of the rectum (*4*), and that the anal canal at this level is adherent to the sphincters (*5*). Waldeyer's fascia (*6*) and the posterior wall of the lateral fascial wings (*7*) are clearly visible at this stage. The simplest way of dissecting out the rectum is to divide Waldeyer's fascia in the posterior midline.

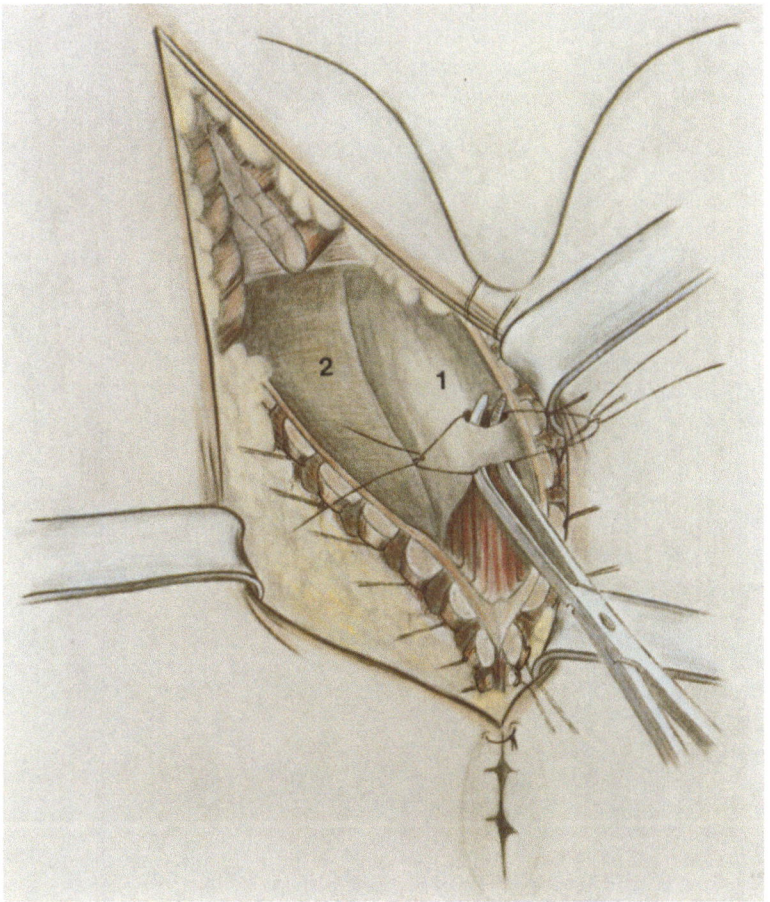

Fig. 20. Waldeyer's fascia (*1*) is incised in the midline with a scalpel and under-mined cranially and caudally through the incision. Between sutures, the incision is extended in stepwise fashion to the lower extremity of the fascia and as far upward as possible. If a pathological adhesion has formed between Waldeyer's fascia and the rectum, division of the fascia is started cranial and caudal to the site of the adhesion.

Occasionally it may be necessary to resect some enclosed perirectal tissue along with Waldeyer's fascia. For this the lateral wings (*2*) and their neurovascular contents must be incised or divided. By proceeding cautiously and keeping as close to the rectum as possible, the surgeon should have no difficulty reaching Denonvillier's fascia on the anterior side and developing a plane of dissection between the posterior surface of this fascia and the rectum.

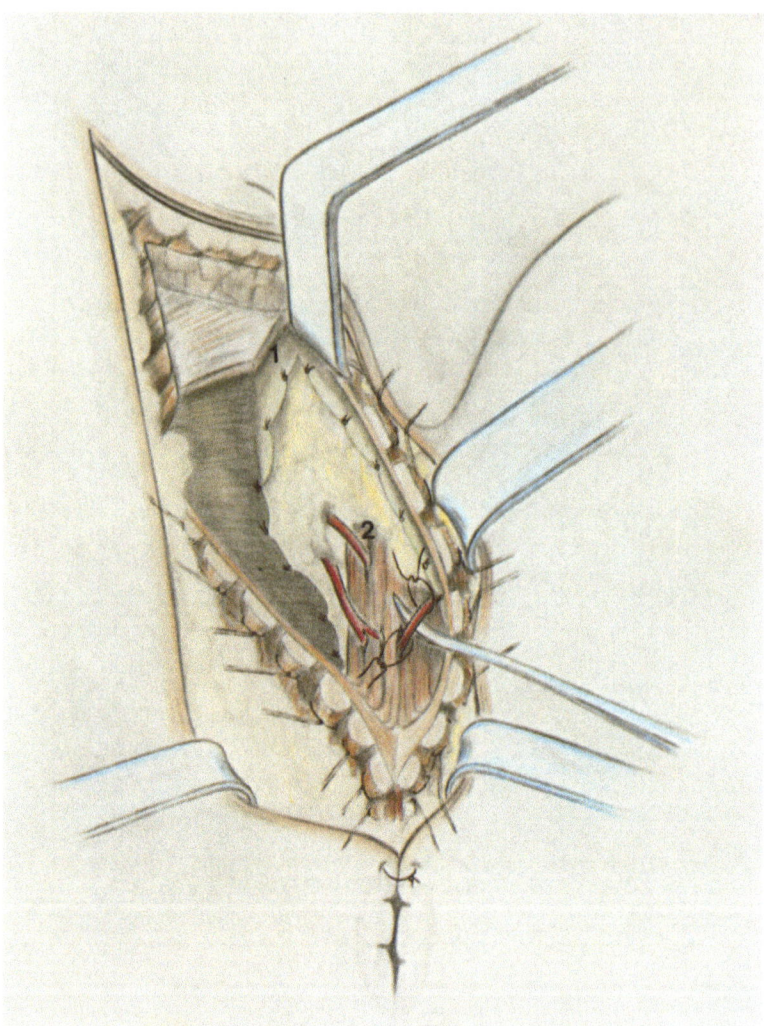

Fig. 21. Waldeyer's fascia can be opened further proximally by notching the sacro-spinous ligament (*1*). After the blood vessels (*2*) and nerves entering the rectum have been divided between ligatures, the rectum can be fully mobilized within its fascial capsule. Because the vascular trunks, ureters, prostate and vagina are located outside the capsule, they cannot be injured by this maneuver.

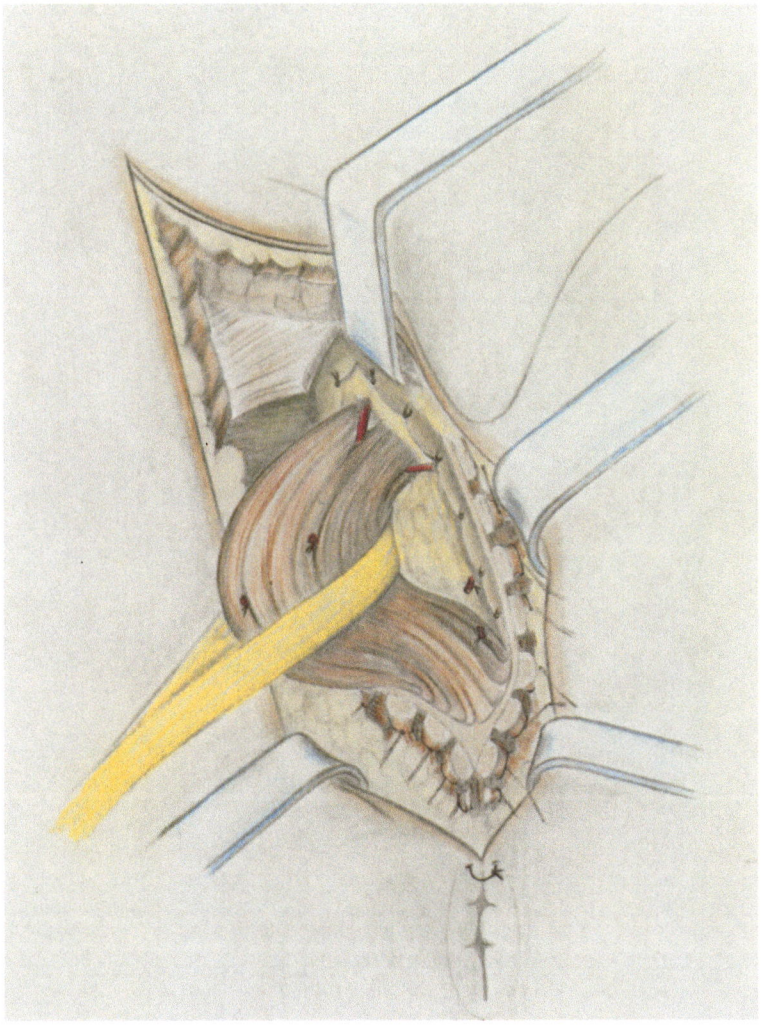

Fig. 22. The rectum is circumferentially exposed and snared. If the disease is localized in the rectum, a proctotomy is performed at this time. It can then be decided whether additional cranial mobilization of the rectum is required (see Fig. 24). In cases of rectal prolapse, a proctotomy is unnecessary, and the rectum is resected about 2 cm above the levator ani. The remainder of the procedure then corresponds to Fig. 24.

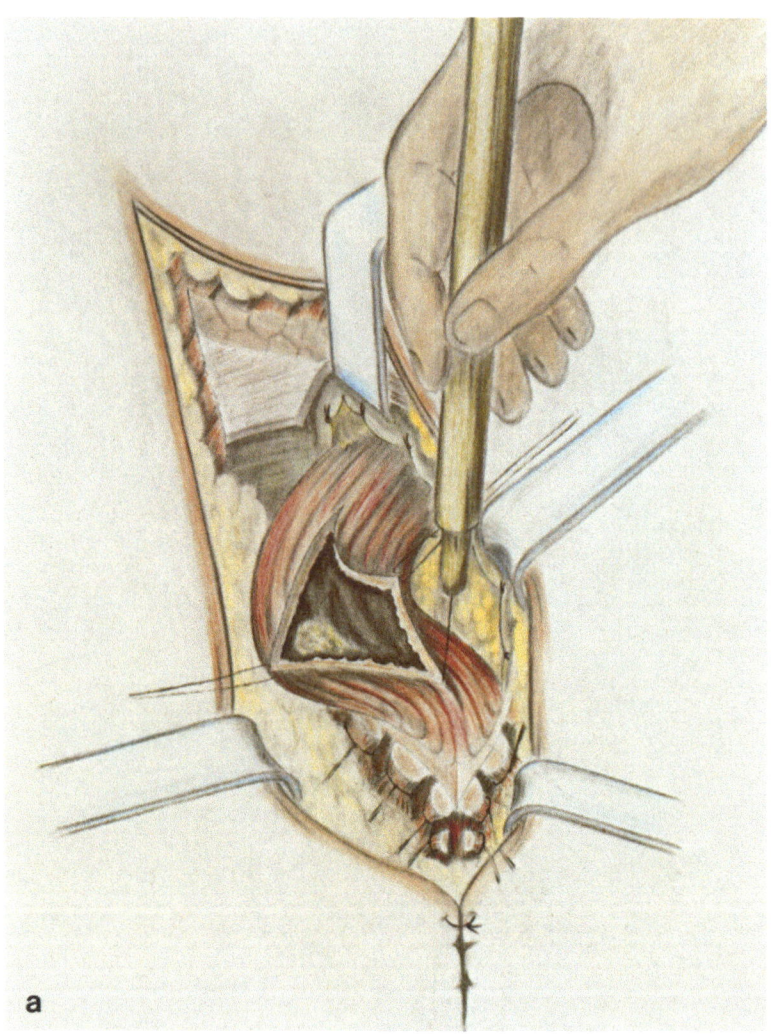

Fig. 23a–e. The rectum is opened longitudinally between stay sutures (**a**). The lumen of the bowel is cleansed with a tissue-compatible antiseptic solution. A growth on the anterior wall of the rectum is easily recognized at this time. Benign tumors are curable by local resection. This is done by making a transverse elliptical excision about the tumor which includes a margin of normal mucosa (**b**). The mucosal defect is closed transversely with simple interrupted sutures (**c**). If a malignancy is present, then a sleeve resection is indicated (**d**). A clearance of

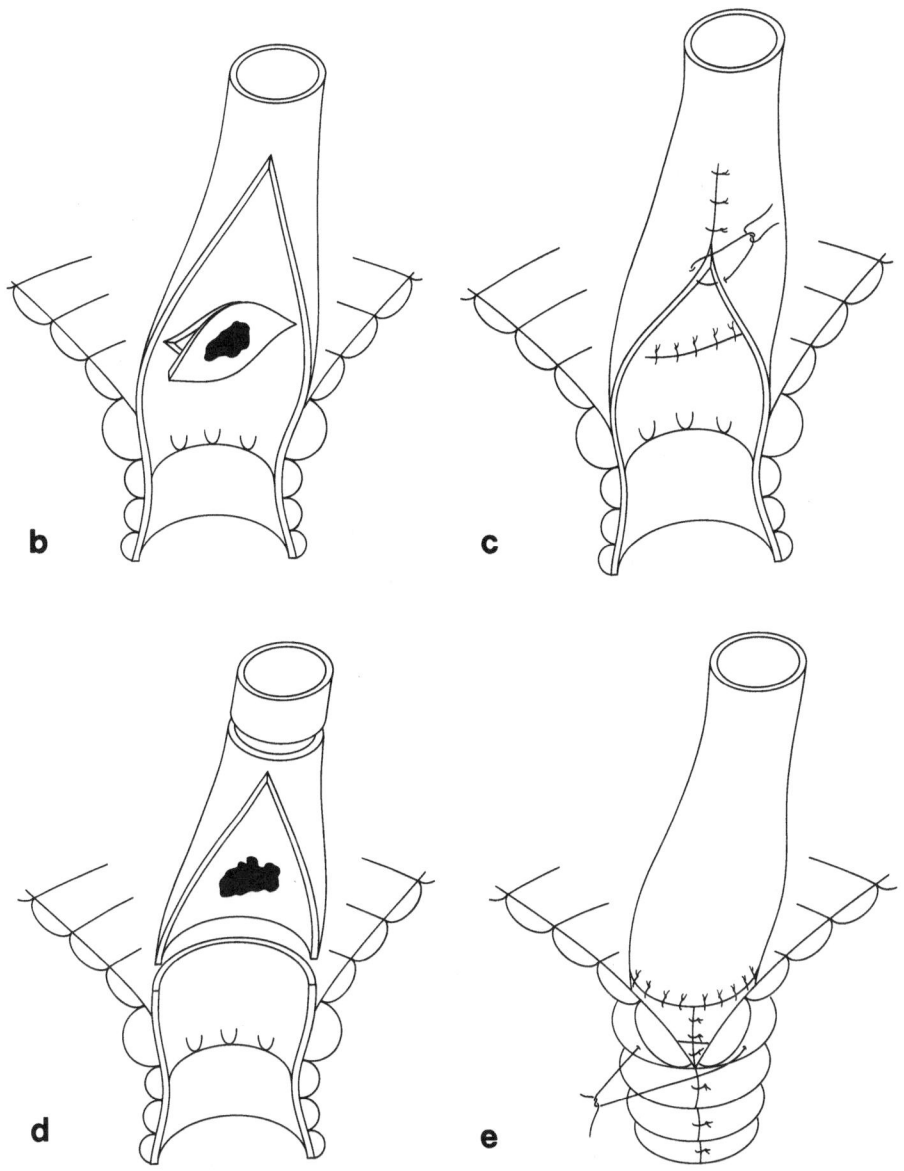

at least 2 cm should be left between the tumor and the cut edges, and a frozen section examination should be done to check the margins of the excised specimen for tumor involvement. If the site and extent of the tumor require more extensive mobilization of the rectum, the surgeon should proceed as in Fig. 24. If the tumor has gone beyond stage Ia + b (TNM classification, UICC 1978) and there is no special indication for a local excision with this technique, it will be necessary to modify the operative plan. The T-shaped suture line created by anastomosis of the bowel ends is illustrated (*e*).

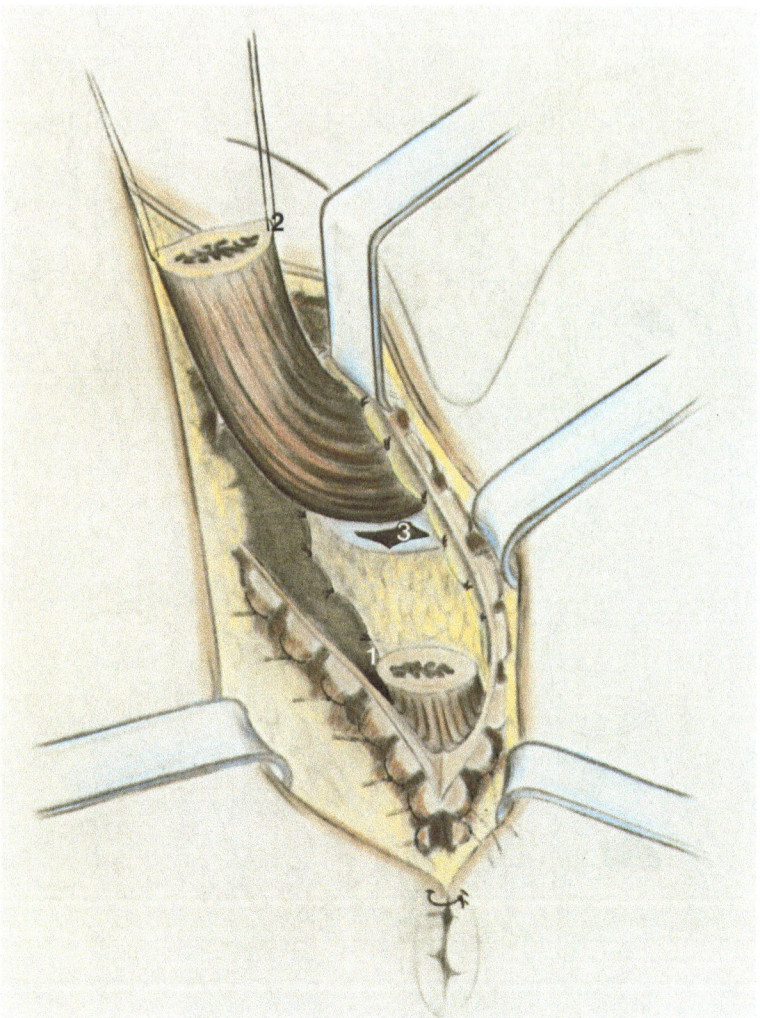

Fig. 24. Depending on the site and extent of the lesion, and in cases of rectal prolapse, it may be necessary to mobilize the rectum further cranially. This is best accomplished by dividing the rectum just above the levator ani (*1*). The lumina of the bowel are cleansed with a tissue-compatible antiseptic solution. The cranial stump (*2*) is snared and may be retracted upward to facilitate anterior dissection. The rectouterine or rectovesical pouch will be encountered and may be opened without concern. Through the opened peritoneum (*3*) the rectum can be traced cranially and mobilized. Segments of prolapsed rectosigmoid up to 35 cm long can be resected in this fashion.

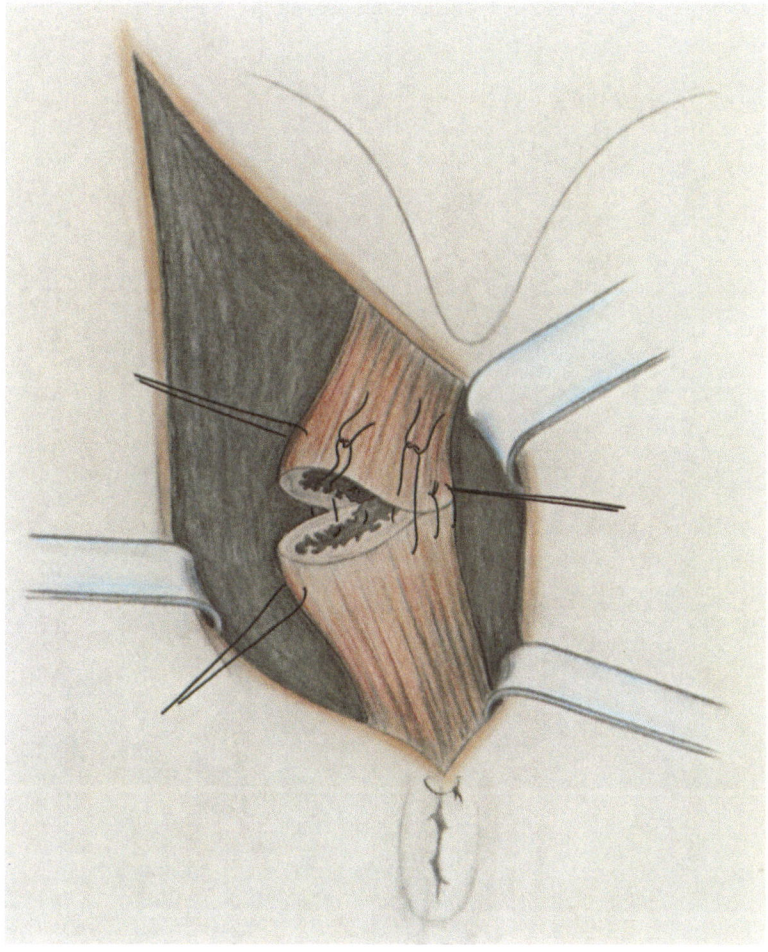

Fig. 25. An end-to-end anastomosis of the bowel stumps is performed according to the general rules of colonic surgery (Hell and Allgöwer 1976), i.e., without tension and in healthy tissue. The sutures must not cut into the tissue. The anastomosis is started in the anterior midline using vertical mattress sutures, and the posterior wall is closed with (sero)muscular sutures. Afterwards the entire wound area is carefully irrigated. The opened peritoneum may be sutured or left open.

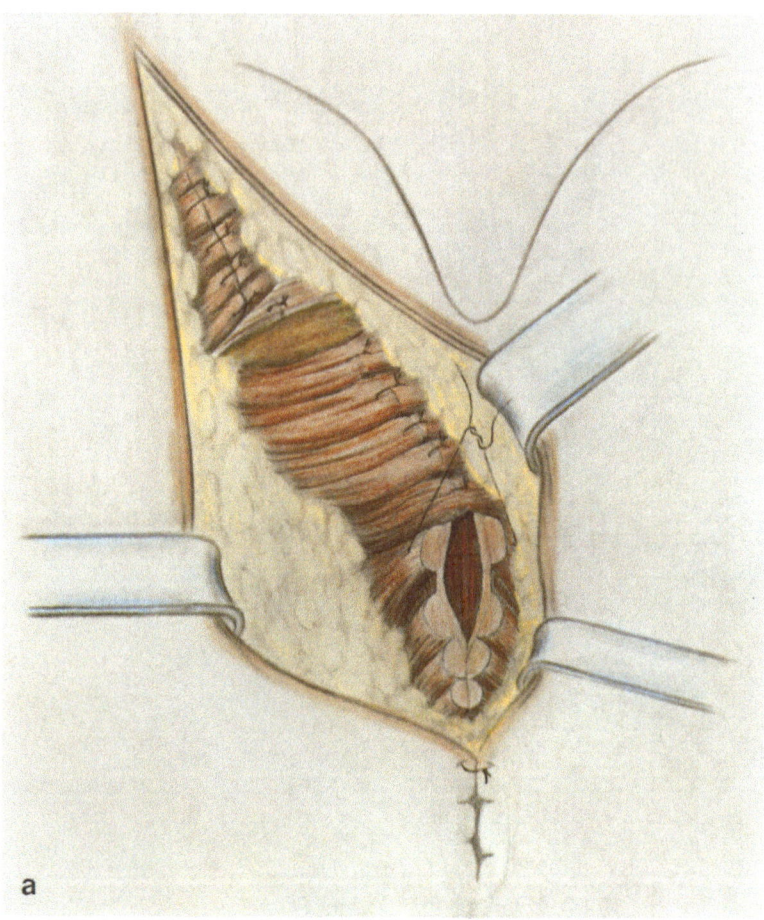

Fig. 26. a For wound closure, the tapes retracting the buttocks are cut. The tagged edges of the levator and sphincter muscles are reapproximated and sutured in sequence. The identifying sutures (not drawn) are left in place. At this time one may elect to reef certain muscles, especially the puborectalis sling, if circumstances require it (e.g., rectal prolapse). If not done previously, a posterior release may now be performed to decrease the anorectal angle. The inner longitudinal

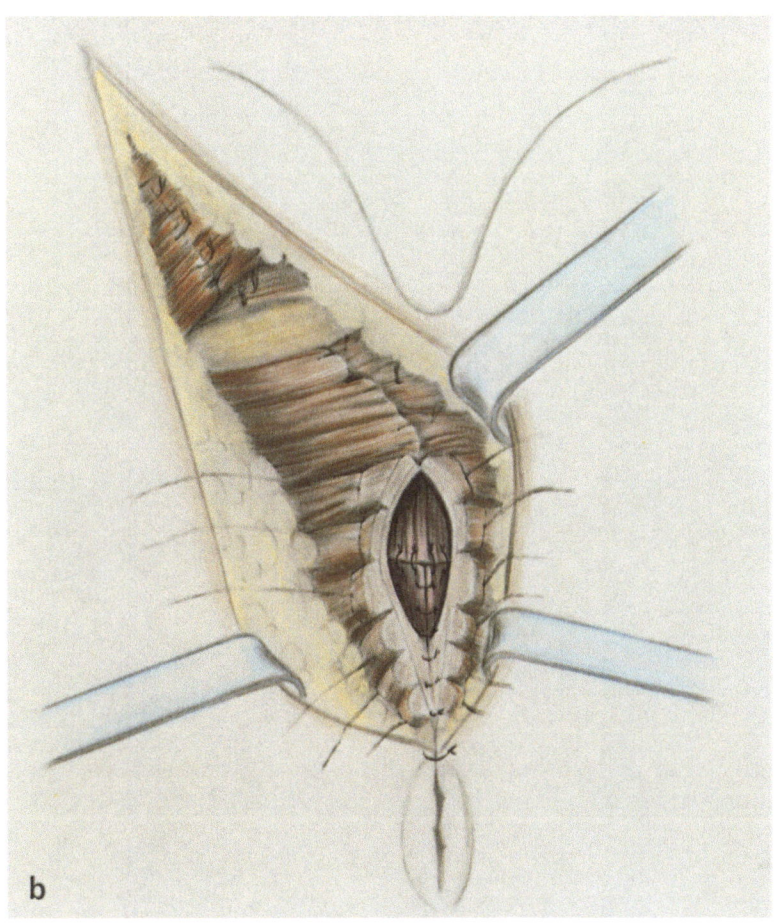

fibers and the fascia of the superior pelvic diaphragm should be included in the sutures. One drain is placed inside and one outside the pelvic floor, and these are brought out through the skin as anteriorly as possible.

Fig. 26. b The T-shaped anastomosis is shown. The skin is closed with vertical mattress sutures.

Part IV
Results and Discussion

At the Surgical Clinic of the Kantonsspital Basel, Switzerland, a total of 81 rectal operations using the parasacral approach were performed between January, 1974, and June, 1982. The indications for these operations are listed in Table 1. The patients ranged in age from 22 to 90 years, with an average age of 65 years. No operative deaths occurred. Nineteen patients developed postoperative wound infections, including superficial disturbances of wound healing. All but two of these resolved completely, leaving no permanent fistulae or incontinence. Two patients developed complete incontinence as a result of their infection and required a permanent colostomy. Since we have instituted preoperative orthograde intestinal lavage and perioperative antibiotic prophylaxis on a routine basis, the incidence of infection has decreased markedly.

Table 1. Rectal diseases treated by parasacral surgery

Diagnosis	N
Carcinoma	36
Myosarcoma	1
Adenoma	9
Prolapse	23
Fistula	5
Ischemic stenosis	1
Traumatic lesion	4
Klippel-Trenaunay syndrome	1
Malformations	1
Total	81

1. Carcinomas of the Rectum

Low-sited rectal carcinomas (4–12 cm from the anal verge) may be removed by proctectomy or by the continence-saving parasacral route. The choice of the procedure depends mainly on the stage of the disease. The general condition of the patient and his willingness to accept a permanent colostomy must also be considered. It should be pointed out that the results which Madden (1971) achieved with the local excision of rectal carcinomas are just as good if not better than the results of proctectomy, taking into account operative mortality. Madden (1971) also found that the prognosis was significantly worsened by lymph node metastases, regardless of the surgical method employed.

Rectal tumors at UICC stage T_1 (tumor confined to mucosa or submucosa) or T_2 (involvement of muscularis) without lymph node involvement or distant spread (UICC Ia and Ib, II) appear to be a good indication for parasacral resection with curative intent. With stage T_3 or T_4 tumors (extension to adjacent or more distant structures), lymph node metastases are probably present, and so a proctectomy with broad evisceration of pelvic lymph nodes will provide a more radical clearance. However, the relatively high surgical risk of proctectomy should be weighed against the minimal risks of the parasacral resection, especially in elderly patients. If there is widespread tumor infiltration or disseminated disease with distant metastases, other palliative measures such as electroresection, cryodestruction, chemotherapy, radiotherapy, or a simple diversion colostomy should be considered. If palliation is the sole intent, the preservation of continence becomes a major concern.

Mason (1974) has devised a system of pretreatment clinical staging based upon the digital assessment of tumor mobility:

Clinical stage I:
The tumor is mobile relative to the rectal wall.
Probable correlation: $T_1N_0M_0$, Ia (UICC 1978).

Clinical stage II:
The tumor is immobile relative to the rectal wall.
Probable correlation: $T_2N_{0-1}M_0$, Ib or III (UICC 1978).

Clinical stage III:
Tumor and rectal mobility are diminished.
Probable correlation: $T_3N_{0-1}M_0$, II or III (UICC 1978).

Clinical stage IV:
The rectum and tumor are fixed.
Probable correlation: $T_4N_1M_{0-1}$, III or IV (UICC 1978).

Clinical stage V:
Disseminated disease.
Probable correlation: $T_{1-4}N_1M_1$, IV (UICC 1978).

In the interests of optimum tumor clearance, the excised specimen should be subjected to a frozen section examination during the operation. Besides allowing intraoperative tumor staging, this technique makes it possible to confirm or exclude involvement of the margins of the resected bowel, enabling the surgeon to judge the adequacy of the resection. Table 2 compares preoperative, clinical assessments of tumor stages in our 36 patients with histologic staging performed during or after surgery. The Table demonstrates the limited reliability of clinical tumor staging and underscores the importance of intraoperative histologic staging.

We feel that the parasacral approach is excellent for the removal of rectal carcinomas at clinical stage I or II (UICC stage Ia or Ib) located between 4 and 12 cm from the anal verge. Resecting these growths together with a sleeve of rectum is curative in a high percentage of cases. For cancers at a more advanced stage, the parasacral approach may still be worthwhile in very old patients or in patients who refuse a permanent colostomy. The advantages of a continence-saving operation, the high risk of proctectomy compared to parasacral surgery,

Table 2. Comparison of preoperative clinical tumor staging with intra- and postoperative histologic staging

Clinical stage (Mason)	N	Postoperative stage (UICC 1978)				
		Ia	Ib	II	III	IV
I	15	7	5	2	1	
II	14		9	1	4	
III	6			1	3	2
IV	1				1	
V	(1)[a]					
Total	36	7	14	4	9	2

[a] Tumor in Mason stage III, but liver metastases present

and the poor prognosis in cases of lymph node metastasis are all factors which influence the operative choice.

The operation (Fig. 27a–d) consists of the following steps:
- Shortly before surgery the bowel is cleansed by orthograde lavage, and prophylactic antibiotics are administered.
- The patient is placed in the Heidelberg position, and the bladder is catheterized.
- Through a left parasacral incision, the pelvic floor muscles are exposed and divided in stepwise fashion; the anal canal is also divided if necessary.
- Waldeyer's fascia is incised in the midline, and the rectum is mobilized; opening pouch of Douglas will facilitate cranial dissection.
- The rectum and anal canal are opened longitudinally between stay sutures; the tumor is evaluated.
- A sleeve of rectum is resected together with perirectal fat (lymph nodes!), leaving at least 2 cm between the tumor and cut edge.
- A frozen section examination is performed on the resected specimen.
- An end-to-end anastomosis is performed using a single layer of 3/0 Dexon. The anterior wall is closed with interrupted vertical mattress sutures tied with the knots inside the lumen, and the posterior wall with simple interrupted sutures tied outside the bowel.
- The divided sphincters and pelvic floor muscles are reapproximated and sutured; the puborectalis sling may be reefed to improve continence.
- Redon drains are inserted without suction; pouch of Douglas is left open; the wound is closed.
- The patient is ambulated as soon after surgery as possible, and oral nutrition is started on the 2nd postoperative day.

Thirty-six patients (22 women, 14 men) underwent parasacral surgery for the removal of a rectal carcinoma. The patients were between 22 and 89 years old, with an average of 61 years.

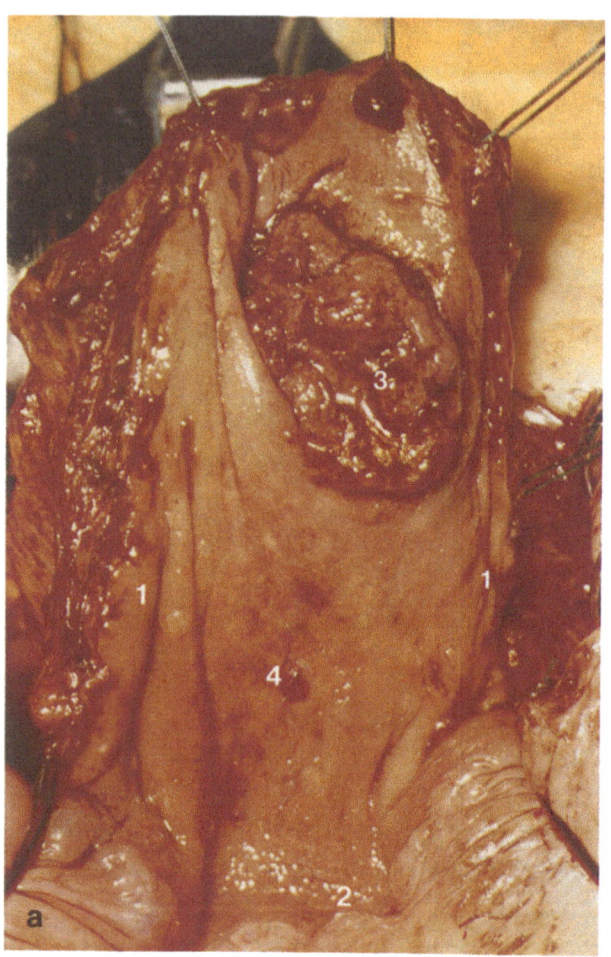

Fig. 27a–d. Resection of a rectal carcinoma.

a (*1*) The anal canal and rectum are opened longitudinally between stay sutures; (*2*) pectinate line; (*3*) carcinoma; (*4*) small adenoma.

b (*5*) The carcinoma in the opened-up, resected sleeve of rectum; (*6*) cranial cut edge; (*7*) caudal cut edge.

c (*8*) The resection edge of the longitudinally-opened anal canal; (*9*) resection edge of the cranial rectal stump.

d (*10*) Anterior continuity restored with vertical mattress sutures tied with knots inside the lumen.

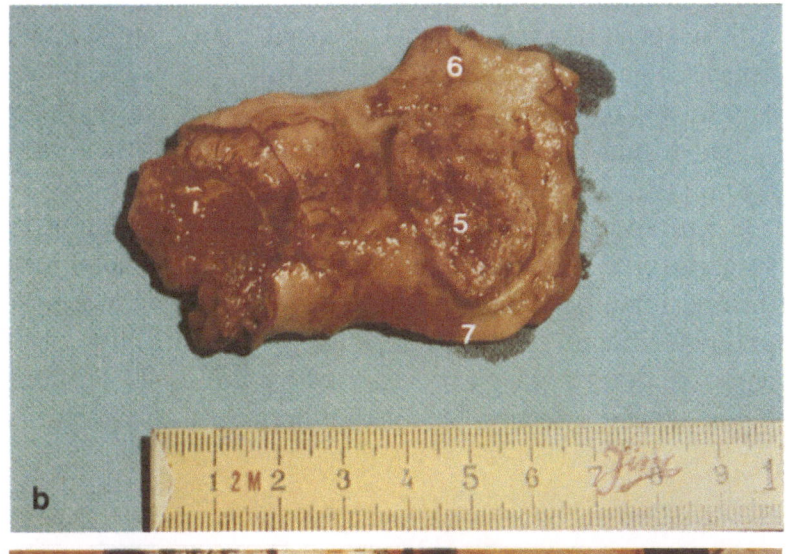

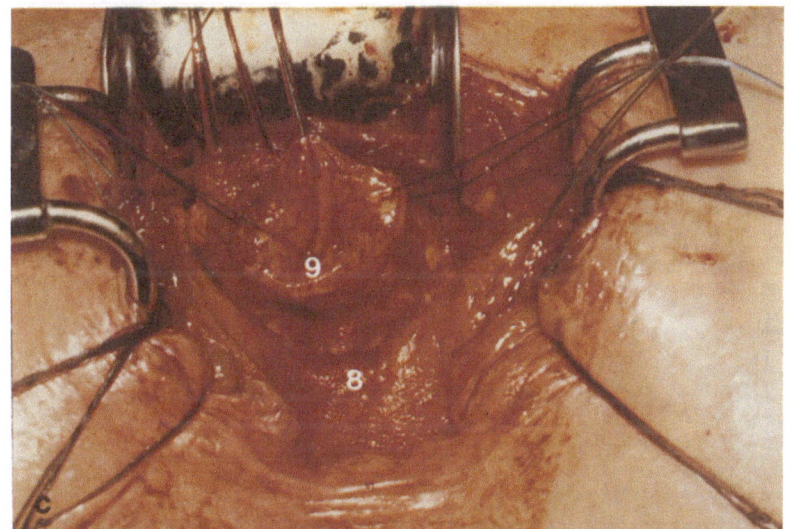

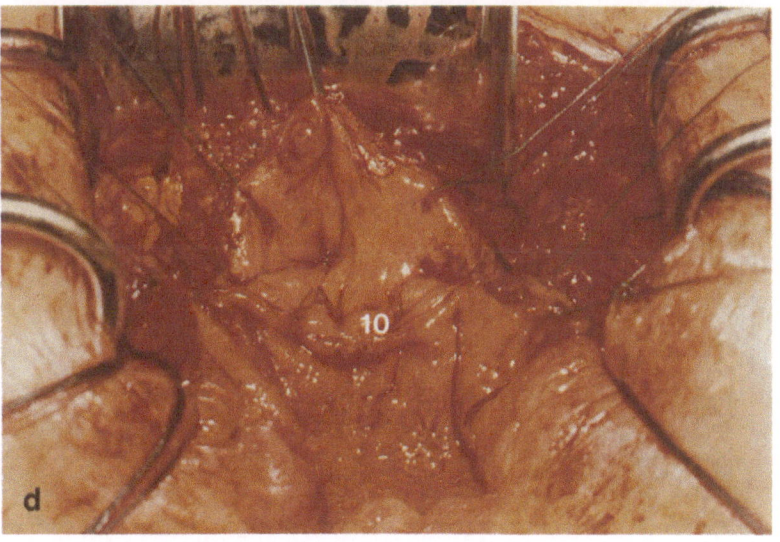

The survival rates after the first operation are shown in Table 3. One patient with a stage III cancer (a 22-year-old man!) and two others with a stage IV cancer categorically refused a colostomy. Autopsy of the stage IV cases disclosed a gastric carcinoma with liver metastases in one of the patients, and a diffuse spread within the pelvis and peritoneum in the other. No local recurrences were found in either case, however.

Recurrences are surveyed in Table 4. In one of the nine patients who underwent surgery for a recurrence, the lesion was located some distance from the site of the anastomosis, and so the growth was identified as a secondary carcinoma.

Eight patients developed a local wound infection, which in four cases was cured by a temporary protective colostomy or by feeding an "astronaut" diet. None of these infections resulted in permanent fistula formation or incontinence.

Table 3. Survival rates after primary operation

UICC stage	N	Living				Dead			
		Time in months							
		6	12	24	36 or more	6	12	24	36 or more
Ia	7	2			5				
Ib	14		2	4	8				
II	4		2	1			1		
III	9		1		2		2		4
IV	2					2			
Total	36	2	5	5	15	2	2	1	4

Table 4. Tumor recurrences

UICC stage	N	Months after first operation				No R	Total R
		6	12	24	36		
Ia	7					7	0
Ib	14	1	1			12	2
II	4		1	2		1	3
III	9	2		2		5	4
IV	2					2	0
Total	36	3	2	4	0	27	9[a]

[a] Of the 9 recurrences, 7 were treated by abdominoperineal proctectomy and 2 by additional parasacral resection

2. Benign and Premalignant Tumors of the Rectum

Benign tumors of the rectum which cannot be radically removed by the transanal route are an ideal indication for parasacral resection. This particularly applies to the villous adenoma, which often forms an extensive, carpet-like growth on the rectal mucosa and may or may not be benign throughout. Usually these tumors can be removed completely and easily owing to the broad exposure of the rectal interior. This approach is also advantageous for the removal of broad-based polyps, for the possibility of malignancy, especially at the base, warrants a really complete excision of these growths. The rare benign neoplasm, such as a hemangioma in the setting of Klippel-Trenaunay syndrome, can also be removed by the parasacral approach without risk and without major blood loss owing to the excellent exposure that is obtained.

The operation consists of the following steps:
- Shortly before surgery the bowel is cleansed by orthograde lavage, and prophylactic antibiotics are administered.
- The patient is placed in the Heidelberg position, and the bladder is catheterized.
- Through a left parasacral incision, the pelvic floor muscles are exposed and divided in stepwise fashion; the anal canal is also divided if necessary.
- Waldeyer's fascia is incised in the midline, and the rectum is mobilized; opening pouch of Douglas will facilitate cranial dissection.
- The rectum and anal canal are opened longitudinally between stay sutures, according to the extent of the pathology.
- The tumor is removed by submucosal resection or elliptical excision.
- An end-to-end anastomosis is performed using a single layer of 3/0 Dexon. The anterior wall is closed with interrupted vertical mattress sutures tied with the knots inside the lumen, and the posterior wall with simple interrupted sutures tied outside the bowel.
- The divided sphincters and pelvic floor muscles are reapproximated and sutured; the puborectalis sling may be reefed to improve continence.
- Redon drains are inserted without suction; pouch of Douglas is left open; the wound is closed.
- The patient is ambulated as soon after surgery as possible, and oral nutrition is started on the 2nd postoperative day.

To date, 9 patients (3 women and 6 men) at our hospital have undergone parasacral surgery for a villous adenoma of the rectum. Their ages ranged from 49 to 77 years; the average age was 66 years. One patient suffered a recurrence one year after the first operation. The growth was resected with a diathermy loop and did not recur. One patient developed a wound infection which healed without complications. All patients acquired full continence postoperatively.

3. Rectal Prolapse

Rectal prolapse is frequently accompanied by partial or complete incontinence, and we feel that it is a good indication for the parasacral procedure. The goal of surgery is to prevent the bowel from prolapsing and, if necessary, to restore anal continence. The parasacral resection of the prolapsed rectosigmoid segment (sliding hernia!) enables simultaneous reconstructive surgery to be done on the incompetent pelvic floor muscles. This consists in detaching the levator from its origin on the sacrum (posterior release) and in reefing the puborectalis sling and external sphincters. These measures help to improve postoperative continence by decreasing the anorectal angle.

The operation consists of the following steps:
- Shortly before surgery the bowel is cleansed by orthograde lavage, and prophylactic antibiotics are administered.
- The patient is placed in the Heidelberg position, and the bladder is catheterized.
- Through a left parasacral incision, the pelvic floor muscles are exposed and divided in stepwise fashion, and the levator is released from its origin on the sacrum.
- Waldeyer's fascia is incised in the midline, and the rectum is mobilized; this is facilitated by opening pouch of Douglas, which is usually quite deep.
- The rectosigmoid segment is resected, the extent of the resection depending on the length of the prolapse.
- An end-to-end anastomosis is performed using a single layer of 3/0 Dexon. The anterior wall is closed with interrupted vertical mattress sutures tied with the knots inside the lumen, and the posterior wall with simple interrupted sutures tied outside the bowel.
- The divided sphincters and pelvic floor muscles are reapproximated and sutured, and the puborectalis sling is reefed.
- Redon drains are inserted without suction; pouch of Douglas is left open; the wound is closed.
- The patient is ambulated as soon after surgery as possible, and oral nutrition is started on the 2nd postoperative day.

To date, 24 patients (21 women, 3 men) have been treated for rectal prolapse at our hospital using this operative technique. They ranged in age from 32 to 90 years, with an average age of 65 years. Only four of the patients were continent prior to surgery. Seven had a relative incontinence, and 13 had complete incontinence. One patient had already had two previous operations for this condition, and another had undergone 13 prior operations of various kinds, none of which had been successful. Following the parasacral operation, there has to date been only one recurrence of a prolapse, which occurred one month postoperatively. The prolapse was reoperated using the same surgical technique, at which time an additional 10 cm of bowel was resected. The patient, a woman, was immediately continent following the second operation. None of the other patients has had a recurrence, including the two patients who had undergone prior operations

Table 5. Follow-up times after parasacral surgery for rectal prolapse

0	Years					
	5	4	3	2	1	<1
Patients	13[a]	2	2		2	3[b]

[a] Two have a permanent colostomy
[b] One had a recurrence of the prolapse

Table 6. Anal continence following parasacral surgery for rectal prolapse

Continence	Number of patients
Complete	11
Improved and satisfactory	7
Unchanged (relatively continent)	4[a]
Worse (incontinent)	2[b]

[a] One had a recurrence after 1 month
[b] Both have a permanent colostomy

(cf. Table 5). Eleven patients became fully continent, and an improved, satisfactory degree of continence was achieved in seven. In four patients continence was not improved by the surgery. The two remaining patients, both women, developed wound infections resulting in a major defect of continence, and permanent colostomies had to be constructed. Since that time, one of these patients has regained the prerequisites for anal continence, but she has declined closure of her colostomy (Table 6). In all, 7 of the 24 parasacral operations were followed by wound infection. Transitory fistulae with unimpaired continence developed in five of these cases, and incontinence developed in the two cases just described.

Most complications, especially the two infections followed by incontinence and permanent colostomy, occured during our initial use of this operative technique. Once the procedure become routine, serious complications were rare and no further incontinence was observed.

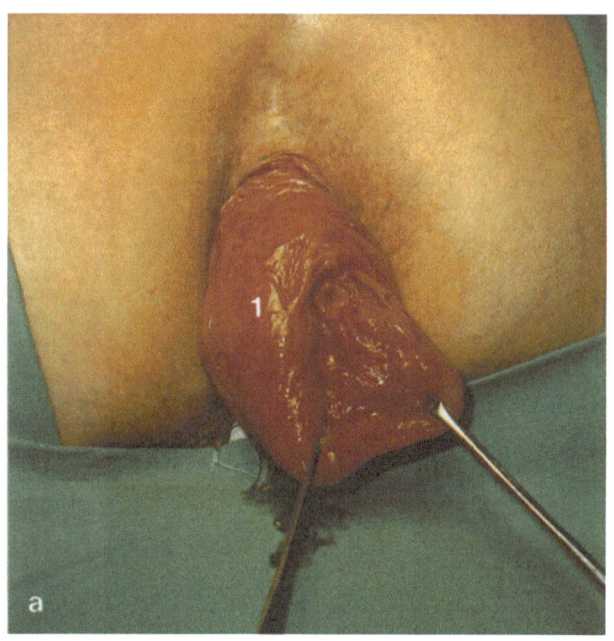

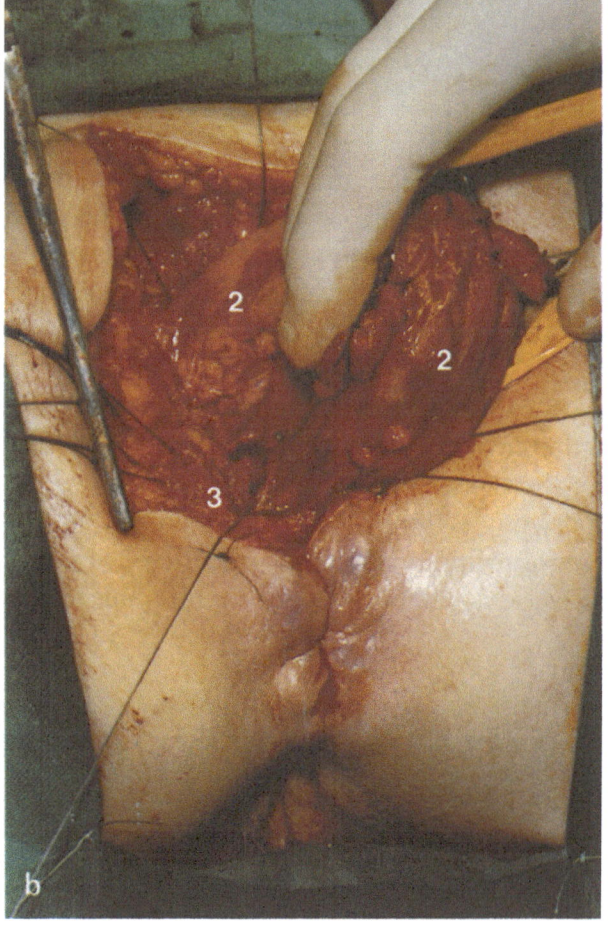

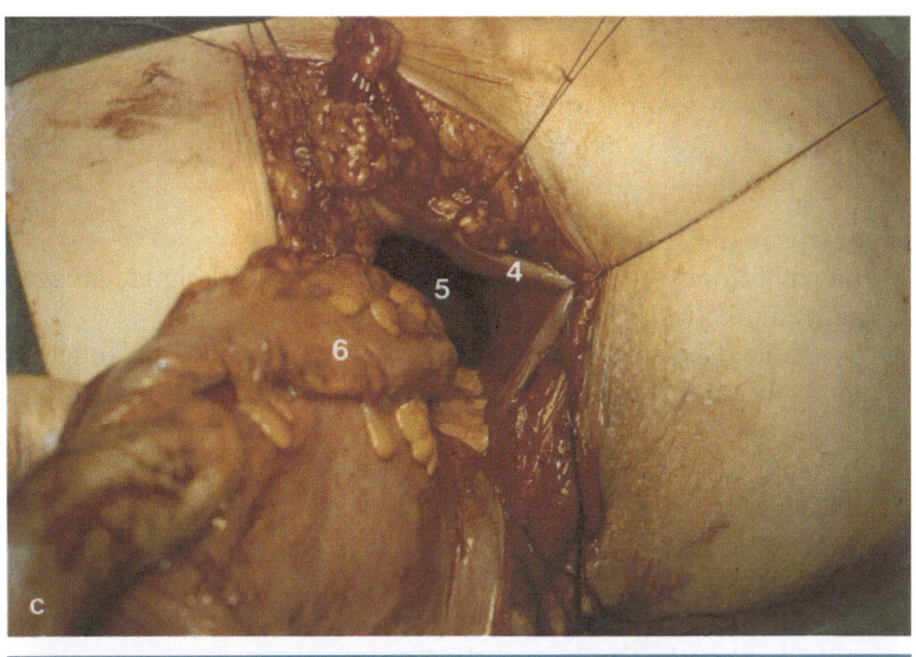

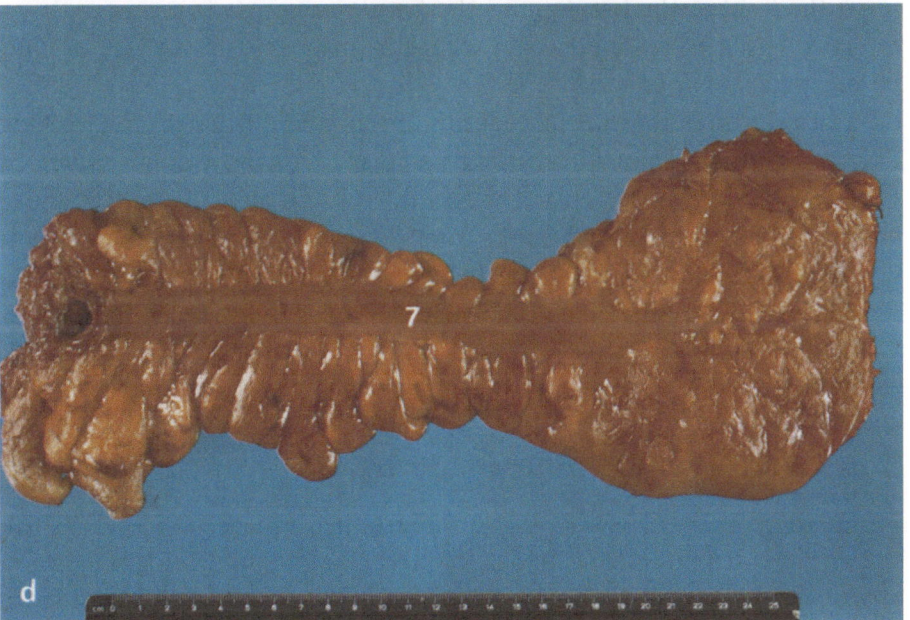

Fig. 28a–d. Resection of a prolapsed rectosigmoid.

a (*1*) Prolapsed rectosigmoid.

b (*2*) Rectosigmoid mobilized through the parasacral approach, according to the length of the prolapse; (*3*) cut edges of the divided levator and sphincter muscles marked with identifying stay sutures.

c (*4*) Peritoneum of opened pouch of Douglas; (*5*) abdominal cavity (Douglas); (*6*) mobilized rectosigmoid.

d (*7*) Resected rectosigmoid (length about 30 cm).

4. Fistulae and Strictures

The parasacral approach is ideally suited for the treatment of high fistulae and cicatricial strictures. Six patients have been operated on for these conditions, with good results.

The steps in the operation are as follows:
- Shortly before surgery the bowel is cleansed by orthograde lavage, and prophylactic antibiotics are administered.
- The patient is placed in the Heidelberg position, and the bladder is catheterized; urethral catheterization may be necessary if organ topography has been altered by scarring.
- Through a left parasacral incision, the pelvic floor muscles are exposed and divided in stepwise fashion.
- Waldeyer's fascia is incised in the midline, and the rectum is mobilized; opening pouch of Douglas will facilitate the dissection.
- The rectum and anal canal are opened longitudinally between two stay sutures at the level of the fistula, and the fistula is exposed.
- The fistula is resected together with any area or segment of bowel showing cicatricial changes.
- Fistulous openings in the rectum and adjacent organs are closed with sutures.
- An end-to-end anastomosis is performed using a single layer of 3/0 Dexon. The anterior wall is closed with interrupted vertical mattress sutures tied with the knots inside the lumen, and the posterior wall with simple interrupted sutures tied outside the bowel.
- The divided sphincters and pelvic floor muscles are reapproximated and sutured.
- Redon drains are inserted without suction; pouch of Douglas is left open; the wound is closed.
- The patient is ambulated as soon after surgery as possible, and oral nutrition is started on the 2nd postoperative day.

Of the five patients who have undergone surgery for rectal fistulae, three had an anorectal fistula, one had a rectovaginal fistula, and one had a rectovesical fistula. One woman was operated on for a cicatricial stricture of the rectum caused by ischemia.

V.G., a 54-year-old man with an extrasphincteric anorectal fistula, was treated by a parasacral fistulectomy. This was followed by uncomplicated wound healing and full continence.

T.A., a 32-year-old man with an anorectal fistulous abscess secondary to proctocolectomy and ileoanostomy for Crohn's disease, was treated by parasacral fistulectomy, additional resection of the anorectal stump, and the creation of a new ileoanostomy. Uneventful wound healing and full continence ensued.

M.B., a 50-year-old man with an anorectal fistula and presacral abscess resulting from a deficient anastomosis following a low anterior resection for rectal carcino-

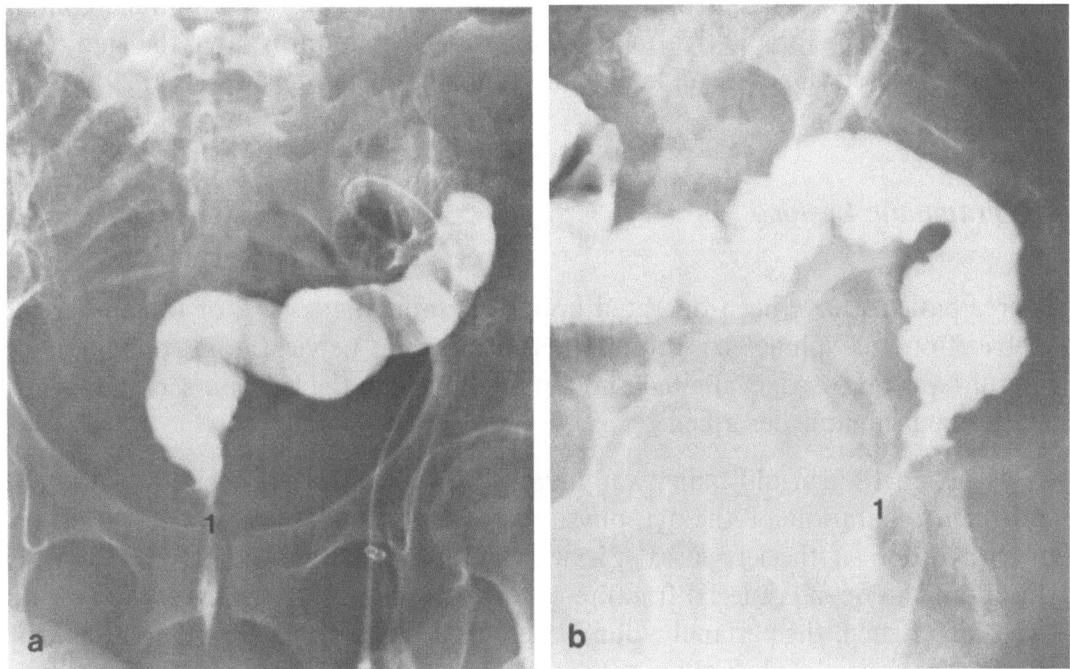

Fig. 29a, b. Visualization of the rectum by barium enema in both the a.p. (**a**) and lateral projections (**b**). (*1*) Stricture of the lower portion of the pars pelvina of the rectum.

ma, was treated by parasacral fistulectomy and drainage. Uneventful wound healing and full continence ensued.

M.E., a 31-year-old woman with a vaginal abscess of unclear etiology and rectovaginal fistulization, was treated by parasacral fistulectomy. Uneventful wound healing and full continence ensued.

P.M., a 60-year-old man with a rectovesical fistula following partial resection of the sigmoid colon for perforating sigmoid diverticulitis, was treated by parasacral fistulectomy. Uncomplicated wound healing and full continence followed. One year later the rectovesical fistula recurred, but so far no secondary operation has been undertaken.

U.H., a 39-year-old women with a large bowel obstruction caused by a rectal stricture, underwent an emergency double-barreled sigmoidostomy. The rectal segment involved by the stricture was resected through the parasacral approach, and the sigmoid was anastomosed to the 3-cm-long anorectal stump. Histology revealed an ischemia-induced cicatricial stenosis with complete destruction of the mucosa. The lesion was attributed to the long-term abuse of ergotamine-containing suppositories for the treatment of migraine. Six months later the sigmoidostomy was closed. Uneventful healing and full continence ensued (Fig. 29a, b).

5. Traumatic Lesions

Three patients have been operated upon for traumatic lesions of the anorectum, pelvic floor or sphincters. Injuries permitting, the pelvic floor, sphincters and rectum were exposed, evaluated and repaired through the left parasacral approach using the technique described.

M.A., an 18-year-old male, was involved in a motorcycle accident, sustaining an open separation of the symphysis, an open grade-III sacroiliac dislocation with avulsion of the left sacral plexus, lacerations of the anorectum and pelvic floor, and an open grade-III fracture of the femoral shaft. A transverse colostomy was constructed, the perianal wounds were inspected and debrided, and the femoral fracture was plated. Eight months later manometry showed sphincter incompetence, and the patient was incontinent (unable to retain an enema). Six months later a parasacral exploration and reconstruction was undertaken, at which time the puborectalis sling was reefed and a posterior release was performed. Two months later manometry of the anorectum showed a marked pressure rise in response to voluntary contraction, and the patient was continent (able to retain an enema). Six months later the patient had virtually normal defecation and complete continence (Fig. 30a, b).

S.H., a 77-year-old man, developed a progressive and finally complete fecal incontinence following an Eisenhammer sphincterotomy for hemorrhoids. He also developed urinary incontinence secondary to a prostatectomy. We attempted to restore continence by reefing the sphincters and puborectalis sling and by performing a posterior release through the parasacral approach. Wound healing was uneventful, and complete fecal continence was regained.

Fig. 30a, b. Traumatic injury of the rectum.   ▷

a Caudal view of the lacerated pelvic floor and perineum with the patient still in the supine position. (*1*) Traumatically exposed, lacerated rectum; (*2*) anus; (*3*) badly-damaged, partially-avulsed left sacral plexus.

b Manometric curves of the anorectum. (*4*) 8 months after primary treatment: squeeze pressure 15 cm H_2O (1.47 kPa) 3 cm from anus, incontinence. (*5*) 13 months after primary treatment: squeeze pressure 25 cm H_2O (2.45 kPa) 3 cm from anus, incontinence. (*6*) 2 months after parasacral exploration and reconstruction (17 months after primary treatment): squeeze pressure 65 cm H_2O (6.37 kPa) 3 cm from anus, full continence.

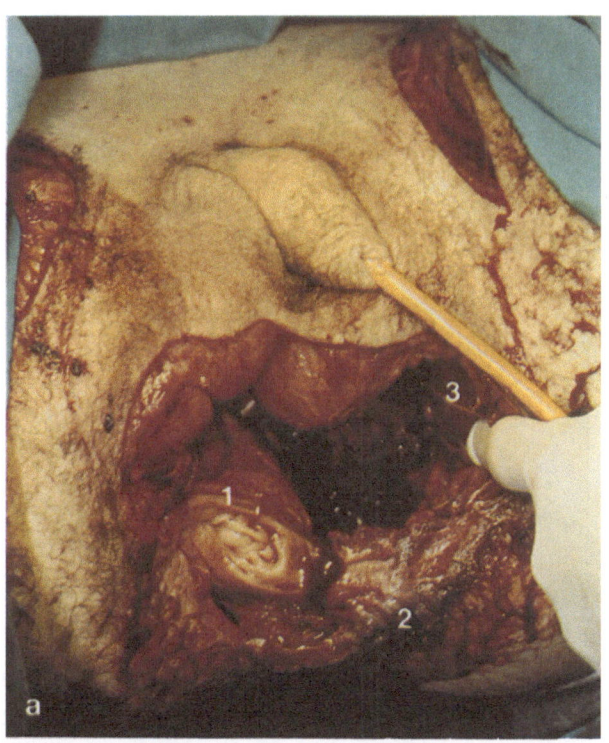

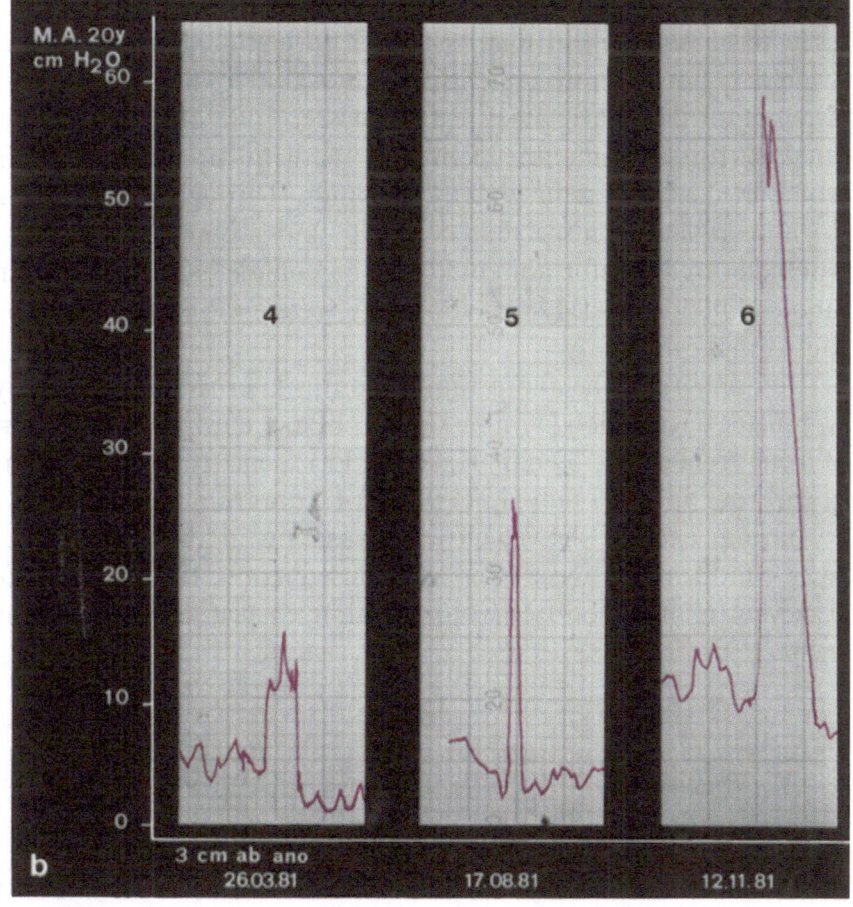

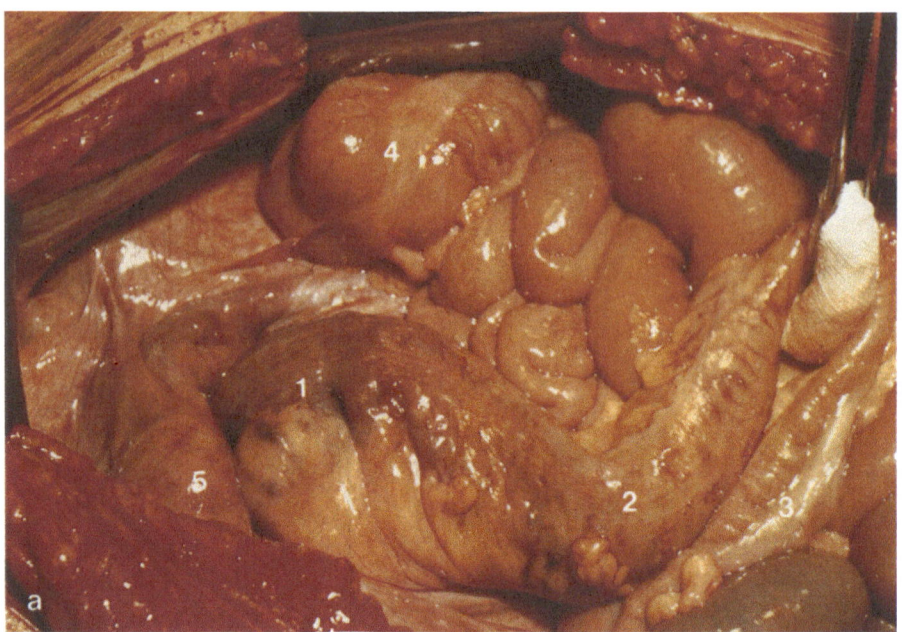

Fig. 31 a–c. Hemangiomatosis of the rectosigmoid. *a* Abdomen at operation. (*1*) Rectum; (*2*) sigmoid colon; (*3*) descending colon; (*4*) cecum; (*5*) uterus.

O.W., a 59-year-old man, suffered an impaling injury of the anorectum and waited 38 hours before presenting for hospital treatment. There was inflammatory swelling of the right gluteal region and scrotum, and palpation disclosed a trans-anal perforation into the perirectal fat with air emphysema in the pelvirectal compartment and right gluteus maximus. Through the parasacral approach the torn rectum was inspected, debrided and sutured. Lacerated portions of the sphincter and levator ani could not be completely repaired. Pararectal drainage and a double-barreled sigmoidostomy were established. The wound healed without complications.

Manometry of the anorectum 3 months later showed relatively poor voluntary sphincter contraction [17 mm Hg (2.3 kPa) 4 cm from anus; 24 mm Hg (3.2 kPa) 3.5 cm from anus; 39 mm Hg (5.2 kPa) 3 cm from anus; 34 mm Hg (4.5 kPa) 2 cm from anus; 37 mm Hg (4.9 kPa) 1.5 cm from anus].

Barium enemas showed no extravasation in the anorectum, and the patient was continent for these enemas. Consequently, the sigmoidostomy was closed. Uneventful, infection-free wound healing ensued, and the patient was fully continent.

6. Malformations

The use of the parasacral approach for the surgery of malformations is illustrated by the case of a 21-year-old woman with hemangiomatosis of the rectosigmoid.

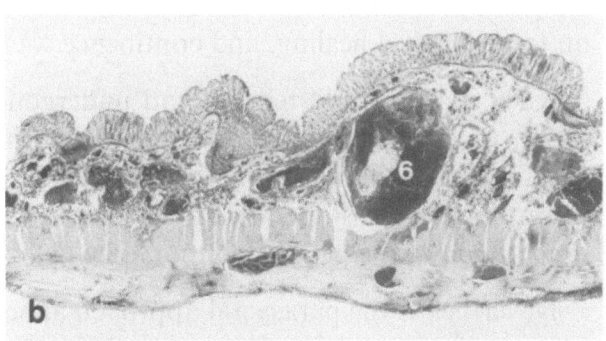

Fig. 31. b Histology of the
resected specimen.
(*6*) Ectatic blood vessels.

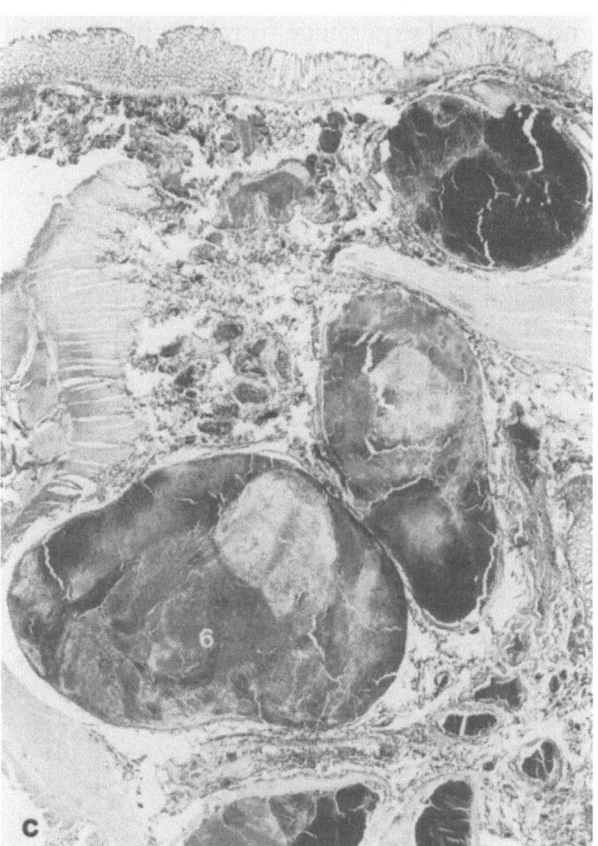

Fig. 31. c Histology of the
resected specimen.
(6) Ectactic blood vessels.
(Photo and evaluation by
M.J. Mihatsch, M.D.,
Institute for Pathology,
University of Basel).

The patient, K.H., a 21-year-old woman, had Klippel-Trenaunay syndrome with typical macrosomia of the right leg and recurrent anal bleeding. Endoscopy revealed marked hemangiomatosis of the rectosigmoid with smaller hemangiomas in the descending colon. A laparotomy was performed, and the left hemicolon was mobilized with sacrifice of the inferior mesenteric artery and middle colic artery. A left hemicolectomy was carried out. The laparotomy was closed, and the patient was turned to the Heidelberg position. At the same sitting the rectosigmoid was resected through the parasacral approach, leaving a 4-cm stump of anorectum. A transversostomy was established. Two weeks later an exploratory laparotomy revealed a left retroperitoneal abscess which was drained. A tempo-anorectum. A transversoanostomy was established. Two weeks later an explora-tory laparotomy revealed a left retroperitoneal abscess which was drained. A temporary abdominal colostomy was constructed. The parasacral wound went on to uneventful healing, and continence was unimpaired (Fig. 31 a–c).

R.F., a 20-year-old female, had undergone a pull-through procedure for anal atresia in childhood. She was completely incontinent when seen at our clinic. A parasacral exploration was undertaken, and a reconstruction of the sphincters was attempted. Postoperatively the patient was still incontinent, and no voluntary innervation of the pelvic floor could be detected.

Nevertheless the parasacral approach appears well suited for the reconstructive surgery of congenital malformations of the anorectum and pelvic floor. We have no personal experience to relate, however, in this area of pediatric surgery.

Bibliography

1. Allgöwer M, et al. (1981) Chirurgische Gastroenterologie. Springer, Berlin Heidelberg New York
2. Bevan AD (1917) Carcinoma of rectum-treatment by local excision. Surg Clin North Am 1:1233–1239
3. Criado F, Wilson T (1981) Posterior transsphincteric approach for surgery of the rectum: The Bevan operation. Dis Colon Rectum 24 (3):145–150
4. Cripps WH (1880) Cancer of the rectum. Churchill, London
5. David VC (1943) The management of polyps occurring in the rectum and colon. Surgery 14:387–394
6. Deucher F (1976) Rund um den Sphinkter: Kontinenzprobleme in der Dickdarmchirurgie. Schweiz Med Wochenschr 106 (9):273–281
7. Dickinson VA (1978) Maintenance of anal continence: a review of pelvic floor physiology. Gut 19:1163–1174
8. Goligher JC (1980) Surgery of the anus, colon and rectum, 4th edn. Baillière Tindall, London
9. Gorsch RV (1941) Perineopelvic anatomy from the proctologist's viewpoint. Tilgman, New York
10. Grant J (1972) Anatomy. Williams & Wilkins, Baltimore
11. Harris LD, Winans CS, Pope CE (1966) Determination of yield pressure: A method for measuring anal sphincter competence. Gastroenterology 50:754
12. Hell K, Allgöwer M (1976) Die Colonresektion. Springer, Berlin Heidelberg New York
13. Holl M (1897) Die Muskeln und Faszien des Beckenausganges. In: Bardeleben K (Hrsg) Handbuch der Anatomie des Menschen, Bd 7. Fischer, Jena
14. Hollinshead W (1971) Anatomy for surgeons, vol 2. Harper & Row, New York San Francisco London
15. Hovelaque A (1927) Anatomie des nerfs craniens et rachidiens et du système grand sympathique chez l'homme. Doin, Paris
16. Ihre T (1974) Studies of anal function in continent and incontinent patients. Scand J Gastroenterol [Suppl] 9:1–64
17. Kerremans R (1969) Morphological and physiological aspects of anal continence and defaecation. Proefschrift voor de graad van geaggregeerde van het hoger onderwijs. Arscia, Brussel
18. Kocher T (1874) Die Exstirpatio recti nach vorheriger Excision des Steißbeines. Zentralbl Chir 10:145–147
19. Kraske P (1885) Zur Exstirpation hochsitzender Mastdarmkrebse. Verh Dtsch Ges Chir 14:464–474
20. Lane R, Parks AG (1977) Function of the anal sphincters following colo-anal anastomosis. Br J Surg 64:596–599
21. Larkin MA (1959) Transsphincteric removal of rectum tumors. Dis Colon Rectum 2:446–451
22. Lawson J (1981) Motor nerve supply of pelvic floor. Lancet (1):999
23. Madden JL (1971) Clinical evaluation of electrocoagulation in the treatment of cancer of rectum. Am J Surg 122:347–352
24. Madden JL (1973) A technique for the performance of an intestinal anastomosis. Surg Gynecol Obstet 136:283–285
25. Martinoli S, Harder F, Allgöwer M et al. (1981) Das Rectumcarcinom. In: Allgöwer M et al. (Hrsg) Chirurgische Gastroenterologie, Bd 2. Springer, Berlin Heidelberg New York, S 797–816

26. Mason AY (1970a) Surgical access to the rectum – a transsphincteric exposure. Proc R Soc Med 63:91–94
27. Mason AY (1970b) The place of local resection in the treatment of rectal carcinoma. Proc R Soc Med 63:1259–1262
28. Mason AY (1972) Trans-sphincteric exposure of the rectum. Ann R Coll Surg Engl 51:320–331
29. Mason AY (1974) Trans-sphincteric surgery of the rectum. Prog Surg 13:66–97
30. Oh C, Kark AE (1972) The transsphincteric approach to mid and low rectal villous adenoma: anatomic basis of surgical treatment. Ann Surg 176:605–612
31. Parks AG, Porter NH, Melzak J (1962) Experimental study of the reflex mechanisms controlling the muscles of the pelvic floor. Dis Colon Rectum 5:407–414
32. Parks AG (1975) Anorectal incontinence. Proc R Soc Med 68:681–690
33. Peham H, Amreich J (1934) Operative gynecology, vol 1. Lippincott, Philadelphia Montreal London
34. Percy J et al. (1981) Electrophysiological study of motor nerve supply of the pelvic floor. Lancet:16–17
35. Pernkopf E (1964) Atlas der topographischen und angewandten Anatomie, Bd 2. Ferner H (Hrsg). Urban & Schwarzenberg, München Berlin
36. Rüedi T, Allgöwer M (1981) Anal- und Rectumprolaps. In: Allgöwer M et al. (Hrsg) Chirurgische Gastroenterologie, Bd 2. Springer, Berlin Heidelberg New York, S 770–775
37. Schärli AF (1981) Über Analyse und Diagnostik von Inkontinenzstörungen. Schweiz Rundschau Med (Prax) 70 (15):656–661
38. Shepherd JJ (1980) Anorectal function. In: Sircus W, Smith AN (eds) Scientific foundations of gastroenterology. Heinemann, London
39. Stephens FD, Smith ED (1971) Ano-rectal malformations in children. Year Book, Chicago
40. Telander RL, Perrault J, Hoffman AD (in press) Early development of the neorectum by balloon dilatation after ileo-anal anastomosis. J Pediatr Surg
41. Toldt C, Hochstetter F (1976) Anatomischer Atlas, Bd 2. Urban & Schwarzenberg, München Berlin Wien
42. Uhlenhuth E (1953) Problems in the anatomy of the pelvis. Lippincott, Philadelphia London Montreal
43. Verneuil AA (1906) A treatise on diseases of the anus, rectum and pelvic colon, 2nd edn. Appleton, New York (Quoted by Tuttle JP)
44. Waldeyer W (1899) Das Becken. Cohen, Bonn
45. Walls EW (1959) Recent observations on the anatomy of the anal canal. Proc R Soc Med [Suppl] 52:85–87
46. Wendell-Smith C, Wilson PM (1977) Scientific foundations of obstetrics and gynecology. In: Philipp E, Barnes J, Newton M (eds) 2nd edn. Heinemann, London
47. Wilson PM (1977) Anorectal closing mechanisms. S Afr Med J 51:802–808
48. Winckler G (1958) Remarques sur la morphologie et l'inervation du muscle releveur de l'anus. Arch Anat Histol Embryol (Strasb) 41:77–95

Subject Index

Colo-Proctology

Editors: **J.-C. Givel, F. Saegesser**

1984. 84 figures, 64 tables. Approx. 190 pages
ISBN 3-540-12557-4

The 1983 Anglo-Swiss Colo-Proctology Meeting, whose proceedings are contained in this volume, enabled numerous specialists to share their experiences in lower gastrointestinal tract pathology. The focus was on ischaemic disease and tumours of the colon, rectum and anus. The articles are written by international authorities in their field, and several contain unpublished results which may lead to new diagnostic and therapeutic methods. Ischaemic lesions are considered in this work because they are far more common than is recognised on clinical grounds alone, particularly in the gastrointestinal tract. Large intestine ischaemia is often confused with other syndromes, especially since the clinical features evoked are, in most cases, atypical. Thus diagnosis is frequently late with dramatic consequences.
The oncology chapter treats basically the early diagnosis of gastrointestinal tumours – a prerequisite for improving survival in affected patients – and also presentation and treatment of certain rare tumours.
The third section of this volume covers diverse subjects such as surgical technique, functional disorders of the large intestine, inflammatory bowel disease, haemorrhoids and investigatory procedures.

Colo-rectal Surgery

Editors: **G. Heberer, H. Denecke**

1982. 91 figures, 89 tables. XI, 204 pages
ISBN 3-540-11505-6

P. Otto, K. Ewe

Atlas of Rectoscopy and Colonoscopy

Translated from the 2nd German edition by B. Clowdus

1979, 124 four-color figures in 21 plates and 31 figures within the text, 1 table. X, 110 pages
ISBN 3-540-09296-X

J. Papillon

Rectal and Anal Cancers

Conservative Treatment by Irradiation – an Alternative to Radical Surgery

Foreword by O.H. Beahrs
1982. 35 figures, 6 color plates. XVI, 201 pages
ISBN 3-540-11626-5

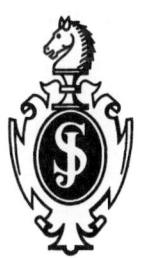

Springer-Verlag
Berlin
Heidelberg
New York
Tokyo

Comprehensive Manuals of Surgical Specialties

Edited by **Richard H. Egdahl**

W. Lawrence Jr., J.P. Neifeld, J.J. Terz
Manual of Soft-Tissue Tumor Surgery
Illustrated by J. Hurd, T. Nicholson
1983. 248 figures in full color, 19 figures in black and white, 43 line drawings. IX, 214 pages
ISBN 3-540-90843-9

E.W. Humphrey, D.L. McKeown
Manual of Pulmonary Surgery
1982. 215 figures (190 figures in full color).
XI, 259 pages
ISBN 3-540-90732-7

Manual of Ambulatory Surgery
Editors: **K.J. Kassity, J.E. McKittrick, F.W. Preston**
Illustrated by J. Koelling
1982. 270 figures (172 figures in full color).
XVIII, 266 pages
ISBN 3-540-90700-9

Springer-Verlag
Berlin
Heidelberg
New York
Tokyo

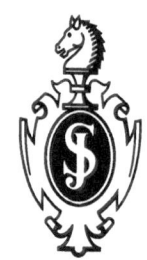

W.P. Longmire Jr., R.K. Tompkins
Manual of Liver Surgery
Illustrated by T. Bloodhart
1981. 230 figures (142 in full color).
XVII, 267 pages
ISBN 3-540-90212-0

B.J. Harlan, A. Starr, F.M. Harwin
Manual of Cardiac Surgery
Volume I
1980. 193 figures (183 in full color), 8 tables.
XV, 204 pages
ISBN 3-540-90393-3

Volume II
1981. 130 figures in full color. XV, 143 pages
ISBN 3-540-90563-4

E.J. Wylie, R.J. Stoney, W.K. Ehrenfeld
Manual of Vascular Surgery
Volume 1
1980. 557 figures, 471 in full color. XII, 264 pages
ISBN 3-540-90408-5

C.E. Welch, L.W. Ottinger, J.P. Welch
Manual of Lower Gastrointestinal Surgery
1980. 215 figures (138 figures in full color),
7 tables. XVI, 276 pages
ISBN 3-540-90205-8

B.J. Masterson
Manual of Gynecologic Surgery
With contributions by K.E. Krantz, W.J. Cameron, J.W. Daly, J.A. Fayez, E.W. Franklin
Illustrator: D. McKeown
1979. 204 figures (192 in color), 12 tables.
XV, 256 pages
ISBN 3-540-90372-0

R.E. Hermann
Manual of Surgery of the Gallbladder, Bile Ducts, and Exocrine Pancreas
With contributions by A.M. Cooperman, C.B. Esselstyn Jr., E. Steiger, R.T. Holzbach
1979. 197 color figures (123 figures in black and white), 16 tables. XIV, 306 pages
ISBN 3-540-90351-8